Design and development of multilayer X-ray optics

Singam Srikanth Panini

List of Figures

List of Tables

Contents

Chapter 1

Introduction

An accidental discovery of X-rays in the year 1895 by Wilhelm Roentgen [Rnt-gen, 1896] is one of the most influential contributions to modern science and technology. These high energy electromagnetic waves quickly revolutionized many diverse areas of scientific research from bio-medical research to experimental quantum mechanics. X-ray astronomy is now a major area of interest in astronomy. Ever since the birth of X-ray astronomy, thousands of celestial bodies are being studied which are emitting X-rays which have revealed fascinating underlying physics.

The region of the electromagnetic spectrum between the Ultra-violet band and Gamma-ray region is classified as X-rays. The wavelength of the X-rays ranges from 0.01 nm to 10 nm. Since X-ray wavelength is very high, X-rays are usually referred in terms of energy. Astronomers classify X-rays into two groups: Soft X-rays (0.1 keV to few keV) and Hard X-rays (few keV to few 100 keV). The energy bands in this classification can slightly vary with applications. Due to absorption of X-rays in the Earth's thick atmosphere, X-rays from celestial bodies do not reach the surface of the Earth. Hence the X-ray astronomical instruments are operated above the Earth's atmosphere using high altitude balloons, sounding rockets and orbiting satellites.

1.1   X-ray emission from astronomical objects

A wide variety of astronomical objects emit X-rays due to several emission mechanisms. The most common mechanism for astronomical X-ray emission is the thermal emission from a very hot object. At temperatures above absolute zero, atoms in material vibrate with the kinetic energy corresponding to the temperature. This allows collisions between atoms and excites electrons to higher energy levels. When the electron decays back to the lower energy level, photons are emitted with the energy corresponding to the difference between two energy levels of electron, which depends on the temperature of the atom. Thermal radiation produces a continuum emission with a peak intensity corresponding to the temperature. Objects at high temperature emit maximum radiation at lower wavelengths. Several astrophysical objects emit X-rays thermally which provides an excellent diagnostic tool to estimate the temperature of the object often hotter than a million degrees.

X-rays are also emitted when a free electron is accelerated around a nucleus of an ionized atom. When a charged particle (say an electron) moves very close to another oppositely charged particle (typically atomic nucleus), the electron gets decelerated/ accelerated emitting electromagnetic radiation. This radiation is called "Bremsstrahlung" radiation or breaking radiation. Another common source of X-rays is synchrotron radiation. Synchrotron radiation process is similar to Bremsstrahlung but the electrons are accelerated by a magnetic field. Astronomical X-ray emission can also be due to inverse Compton scattering when the relativistic electron collides with low energy photons (say Cosmic Microwave Background photons). When an electron with relativistic speed collides a photon, the electron can share part of its energy to the photon to produce X-rays. Inverse

Compton X-ray radiation is commonly seen in supernovae [Woltjer, 1964], [Goren-stein et al., 1970] and Active Galactic Nuclei (AGN) [Liang, 1979]. X-rays are produced by solar system objects like the planets [Metzger et al., 1983], [Bhard-waj et al., 2007], Moons [Giacconi et al., 1962], [Narendranath et al., 2010] and Comets [Cravens, 2000] mostly by fluorescence from the solar X-rays and the charges exchange reactions from ions present in the solar wind.

1.2 Astronomical X-ray sources

1.2.1 Solar and stellar X-ray emission

In stars (including our Sun) X-ray emission is mainly due to the hot outer atmo-sphere, the corona [Frost, 1969], [Rosner and Vaiana, 1980], [Rosner et al., 1985]. The corona ($\sim$ 2 million degree Celsius) is much hotter than the photosphere ($5,500^oC$). Hence, the corona emits thermal X-rays. X-ray spectroscopic study of the Sun and stellar objects provides a better understanding of the corona and its elemental abundances [Doschek, 1990], [Telleschi et al., 2005], [Audard et al., 2001], [Güdel et al., 2001] . These studies also provide a diagnostic to understand the long-standing coronal heating problem [Schatzman, 1949]. Solar and Stel-lar X-ray emission is also associated with dynamic activities like flares [Kundu, 1961], [Cline et al., 1968]. The flux intensity and spectral nature of the X-ray emission change drastically with flares.

1.2.2 Solar system bodies

Solar system bodies are now known to emit X-rays either by fluorescence of plan-etary atmosphere or surface from impinging solar X-rays and charge exchange reactions from the neutral atoms in the atmosphere through interactions with the solar winds [Bhardwaj et al., 2007], [Cravens and Maurellis, 2001], [Maurellis and Cravens, 2001], [Dennerl, 2003] . Both fluorescence and charge exchange reactions produce characteristic line emissions from the elements present in the atmosphere/ surface. X-ray observations of these objects facilitate study the elemental composition in the atmosphere [Branduardi-Raymont, 2011], [Narendranath et al., 2011], [Athiray et al., 2013], [Athiray et al., 2014], [Narendranath et al., 2010].

1.2.3   Supernovae

Supernovae are one the most energetic events in the universe. In core-collapse supernovae (type II, type Ib and type Ic supernovae), the nuclear power source at the center (core) exhausts its energy and the core collapses. This causes the formation of a neutron star or a blackhole (depending on the mass of the initial star). This process releases an enormous amount of energy in the form of radiation, heat and Neutrinos. The remnants of the explosion (except the central neutron star), expands radially out with speed exceeding few tens of millions of kilometers per hour as a thermonuclear shock wave. X-rays are produced by the heat and the shock wave from the supernova remnants [Colgate, 1968], [Schwartz et al., 1972], [Ilovaisky and Ryter, 1972]. Several high atomic number elements are formed during the supernova explosion which can be studied using X-ray observations [Tsunemi et al., 1986], [Ballet and Decourchelle, 2002].

1.2.4   Neutron stars and black holes

Neutron stars and black holes are one of the most fascinating objects in the universe. These are the remnants of a massive star after a supernova explosion. The core of the star collapses due to huge gravitational force. In a neutron star, all matter is converted into a stable neutron gas attaining the density of about $10^{15} g/cm^3$ [Cameron, 1959]. The rotational kinetic energy and the magnetic field of the star prior to the collapse get greatly intensified and transferred to the neutron star. High speed rotating neutron stars intensifies an already strong magnetic field of a neutron star. These are called Magnetars with magnetic fields about $10^{14} - 10^{15}$ Gauss [Duncan and Thompson, 1992]. The rapidly rotating magnetic field of a neutron star accelerates particles to relativistic energies and produces synchrotron radiation emitting broadband electromagnetic radiation from Radio to X-rays [Meltzer and Thorne, 1966], [Bisnovatyi-Kogan and Fridman, 1969]. If a neutron star or a black hole is accompanied by a normal star in a gravitationally bound orbit, the gas from the companion star is accreted by the compact object and forms an accretion disc of gas around it. During the process of accretion, the matter gets heated in the disc and emits thermal radiation. The temperature of the disc increases as the matter flows closer to the neutron star and emits X-rays from inner regions of the disk. These are some of the brightest sources of X-rays in the universe and hence named X-ray binaries. X-ray observations of these objects gives the temperature profile and radiation process from the accretion-powered neutron stars/ black hole.

1.2.5 Galaxies

Galaxy X-ray emission is due to the sum of all X-ray sources like the main sequence stars, neutron stars, supernova remnants, and diffuse gas. Most galaxies have a supermassive black hole in their center. These black holes grow by accretion of matter from the host galaxy and emit X-rays. These are called Active Galactic Nuclei (AGN) and their X-ray emission tends to dominate the total galaxy's X-ray emission. AGNs reach luminosities of $10^{46} erg/s$ [Franceschini et al., 1994] in comparison to the X-ray emission of galaxies of the order 10^{39} to $10^{42} erg/s$. X-ray emission from AGNs is mainly due to the thermal emission from fast-moving matter in the accretion disk [Payne, 1979], [Takahara et al., 1981]. AGNs also produces X-rays from non-thermal radiation from jets in the direction perpendicular to the accretion disk [Cheung, 2004]. AGN jets emit highly collimated synchrotron radiation across the entire electromagnetic spectrum from radio waves to gamma rays.

1.2.6 Galaxy clusters

Galaxy clusters are the largest gravitationally bounded objects in the Universe. Galaxy clusters mainly consist of hundreds of galaxies, vast clouds of hot gas and dark matter. X-ray observations of galaxy clusters indicated that the total X-ray flux of the cluster is significantly higher than the sum of X-ray emissions of individual galaxies [Canizares, 1987]. This excess emission is due to emission from hot gas in clusters. The total mass of hot gas is around 2- 10 times the mass of all galaxies in the cluster [Jones et al., 1979]. The gas in galaxy clusters is heated to about 30- 100 million degrees during cluster formation making it the dominant source of X-rays [Girardi et al., 1996], [Tucker et al., 1998]. The X-ray emission from intergalactic gas can exceed from 10-100 time the total X-ray flux emitted by all galaxies in a cluster. X-ray observations of galaxy clusters help in understanding the cluster formation and evolution.

1.2.7 Gamma Ray Bursts (GRBs)

GRBs are the brightest electromagnetic events so far observed in the known Universe. GRBs are transient events emitting a bright flash of gamma rays in the timescales varying from a few milliseconds to a few minutes [Marar et al., 1981]. Several models are being currently investigated to explain such bright high energy events. Evidence from recent satellites like Swift [Hill et al., 1999] and Fermi [Atwood et al., 2009] indicate that gamma-ray bursts are caused by the collapse of matter into a black hole [MacFadyen and Woosley, 1999]. GRBs produce afterglow at low energies from X-ray to radio waves whose time scales are long enough to track the event [Costa et al., 1997]. X-ray observations of such afterglow can measure the amount of gas in the vicinity of the burst and indicate the elemental composition of the gas [Reeves et al., 2002].

1.3 Astronomical X-ray instruments

Due to absorption of X-rays from Earth's thick atmospheric gases, X-rays from celestial sources do not reach Earth's surface. While this protects life on earth by shielding harmful high energy radiation, makes it impossible to observe celestial objects in X-rays from ground. Hence astronomers use high altitude balloons, sounding rockets and orbiting satellites to send X-ray instruments above the thick atmosphere to observe astronomical X-rays sources. This not only makes astronomical X-ray instrumentation naturally more expensive but also imposes several restrictions on the size and weight of the overall instrument. These constraints along with the fact that most astronomical objects are relatively very faint, has limited progress in the understanding of astronomical X-rays sources and it remains as a major area of research.

1.3.1 X-ray detectors

Most X-ray detectors work on the principle of the photoelectric effect. When an X-ray photon interacts with the detector medium it produces photoelectrons. These electrons are then collected and amplified by electronic circuits which records the time and amplitude of the event. The detector medium can be gas or a semiconductor. Gaseous detectors can be built to provide large effective areas and are very popular in astronomy applications. Historically most of the first generation X-ray instruments are gas based X-ray detectors without any optics.

Proportional counters

Proportional counters are the first generation gas based X-ray detectors but continue to have active applications in the astronomy. These are not only efficient X-ray detectors but can also measure the energy of every X-ray photon detected. A proportional counter consists of a gas (preferably inert gas) sealed with a thin window which form an active area. When X-rays interact with the gas medium, it ionizes gas and produces electrons. These electrons are then collected by an electrode located at the center of the gas medium. Depending on the gas medium, each X-ray photon releases a specific number of electrons resulting from the interaction. The number of electrons produced by the gas is given by the ratio of the X-ray photon energy and the energy required to emit one electron from the gas. Typically a 1 keV photon produces around 30-40 electron-ion pairs. The number of electrons produced by a single photon is proportional to the photon energy. Individual photon events are readout enabling spectroscopic studies. By counting the number of electrons collected by the electrode, one can estimate the energy of the incident photon. Given a gas medium, it is possible to develop very large area proportional counters ($\sim 1000\ cm^2$). A major challenge in developing large area proportional counters lies in maintaining the gas in the detector without any leak. The window on the active area side should be thin so as not to absorb X-rays yet very strong to sustain the vibrations of the rocket launch and not have any pinholes which could result in gas leaks. Several early missions were lost due to the failure of windows during launch. 0.1 mm Beryllium (Be), thin Aluminised mylar or even thin plastic is generally used as a window to a proportional counter detector. Table 1.1 gives the list of some of the earlier astronomical instrument that used large area proportional counters.

Table 1.1: Details of some of the large area proportional counter detector flown for astronomical observations. References: [Giacconi et al., 1971], [Peterson, 1975], [Turner et al., 1981], [Turner et al., 1989], [Bradt et al., 1993], [Yadav et al., 2016]

Experiment	Year	Bandwidth	Area (cm^2)
Uhuru	1970	2-20 keV	2×840
HEAO- A1	1977	0.15-20 keV	7×1350
EXOSAT ME	1983	1.2-50 keV	1800
Ginga LAC	1987	1.5-37 keV	4000
RXTE PCA	1995	2-60 keV	6250
Astrosat- LAXPC	2015	3-80 keV	3×2000

Several techniques can be adapted to make a position sensitive proportional counter. If the anode is made of resistive material, the position of the event along the wire can be determined by the relative size of the pulse measured at the two ends of the wire [Borkowski and Kopp, 1972]. This gives one-dimensional information of the event. The proportional counter can be made with multiple wires to get the event's position information along the perpendicular axis of the wire [Sun and Richardson, 1954]. This type of proportional counters are known as imaging proportional counters or position sensitive proportional counters.

Another mode of operating gas detectors is the gas- scintillation proportional counter [Shamu, 1961]. Instead of detecting the photoelectrons from the event, gas-scintillation proportional counters detect the optical or ultra-violet flashes or scintillations that occur in the gas medium when the ions recombine with electrons. The energy resolution of the detector in this mode is much better than the standard proportional counters.

Scintillation counters

For hard X-rays with energies greater than 20 keV, the quantum efficiency of gas-based proportional counters drops. This is because the gas becomes transparent for high energy X-rays. Hence a high absorbing material is needed for hard X-rays. A scintillation counter uses inorganic crystals like Sodium iodide or Caesium iodide which stops high energy photons up to several MeV [Aitken, 1968]. The crystal attached to a photodiode acts as a scintillation counter. When X-rays impinge on the crystal, optical flashes of light are generated which are recorded by the photodetector. The amount of light produced by scintillation is proportional to the energy of incident photon energy which drives the spectral resolution.

Micro-channel plates

Micro-channel plates (MCPs) are small glass tubes which are treated to enhance emission of secondary electrons when photons are incident. MCPs consist of a photo-cathode typically coated with Caesium Iodide (CsI) to enhance the efficiency of photo-electron generation. Photo-electrons are then accelerated down the tube to the anode by applying large voltages. As they progress, they strike the wall and liberate more electrons. Each primary electron can finally result in as many as 10^8 secondary electrons at the positive end. Due to advancements in the glass fiber technology, the diameter of each tube can be made as small as 10 microns. A typical MCP of 25 mm diameter can give about 3 million individual channels each which act as a pixel to produce a position sensitive image. X-ray missions like the Einstein [Giacconi et al., 1979], ROSAT [Truemper, 1982], and Chandra [Weisskopf et al., 2000] used MCPs for high-resolution imaging.

Solid state detectors

A solid-state device acts as an X-ray detector by collecting the photo-electrons produced by the incident X-ray photon in the material. The working principle is similar to that of a gas-based detector with an exception that the interaction medium is a solid. The major advantage of solid state detectors for space application is that they operate at much lower voltages. Solid state detectors have to be cooled to very low temperatures ($\sim -100^o$ C) to avoid the emission of thermal electrons. As the number of electrons generated by a solid state device is much larger than by gas, the energy resolution of solid state device is much higher than the gas based proportional counters [Soltau et al., 1996]. Due to exponential growth in the semiconductor technology in the recent past, each solid state detector can be made very small (10 microns) and can be placed in arrays of $\sim 10^6$ detectors. These detectors are known as Charge Coupled Devices (CCDs) [Boyle and Smith, 1970] and are widely used in optical astronomy for several decades. Small size, large quantum efficiency, fast readouts and good spectral resolution for single photon readout made CCDs very popular imaging detectors in astronomical X-ray instruments. X-ray missions like Chandra [Weisskopf et al., 2000], XMM Newton [Gondoin et al., 2000], and future missions like eROSITA [Predehl et al., 2007] used CCDs for high-resolution imaging and spectroscopy.

Micro calorimeters

Microcalorimeters are a recent development in X-ray detector technology [Moseley et al., 1985]. The absorbing material in microcalorimeters is maintained close to absolute zero (<0.1 K). When an X-ray photon is incident on the device, the energy in the photon gets transferred to heat and raises the temperature of the medium. This small rise in temperatures can be measured by sensitive thermometers which gives information on the incident photon energy. These devices have a very high spectral sensitivity of the order of a few electron volts (~ 5 eV) [Jach et al., 2009]. Suzaku mission [Kunieda et al., 2006] used microcalorimeter but unfortunately, it couldn't record any scientific data as the refrigerators failed. Hitomi X-rays telescope [Takahashi et al., 2018] used microcalorimeters for soft X-rays spectroscopy. It provided a spectral resolution of about 7 eV at 2 keV. Not much

scientific data are available with this instrument due to a premature shut-down of
the mission after one month from the launch due to an accident while orbiting. Future mission concepts like Hitomi followup-XRIM, Athena [Lotti et al., 2014] and
LynX [The Lynx Team, 2018] propose to use microcalorimeter for high-resolution
spectroscopic studies.

1.3.2 Position sensitive X-ray instruments

X-ray detectors provide good sensitivity to record flux from cosmic point X-rays
sources. However bare detectors can only provide very coarse localization of source
and provide no inputs on morphology/ structure of source. Hence additional front-
end image capturing hardware is required to localize and image the source with
useful spatial resolution. Over the past few decades, front-end instrumentation
has evolved from just localizing the source position over a few degrees to resolving
the spatial features of an extended object of an order of a few arc seconds.

Collimators

One of the simplest technique to localize the source position is to use collimator
in front of the detector. A collimator consists of a physical occulter to restrict
light from large field angles. The field of view is restricted by reducing the width
and increasing the length of the collimator. Field of view of the collimator can
be made small enough that only one bright source on the sky is observed at a
time. In order to finally restrict the field of view. Another variant of collimators
includes Scanning Modulation Collimator (SMC) [Oda et al., 1976]. SMC consists
of one-dimensional wire grids. As the detector scan across the source, the signal is
modulated by the shadow pattern of the grid. SAS-3 [Doxsey, 1975] and HEAO-
1 [Roy et al., 1977] instruments scanning modulator collimators to locate bright
X-ray objects in the sky.

Coded mask

Coded masks work similar to scanning modulation collimators with an exception that the modulation is spatially driven instead of temporal. Implementation of coded mask technique in astronomy was first proposed in 1968 [Ables, 1968] [Dicke, 1968] . A coded mask consists of a 2-d (or 1-d) mask with transmission and absorbing plates arranged in a specific pattern. The mask produces shadow when source photons incident on the mask are parallel, the observed shadow-pattern being based on the relative position of source in mask frame on a two-dimensional position sensitive X-ray detector. A shift in the pattern is directly correlated to the source location on the sky. Several X-ray missions including Uhuru (1970) [Jagoda et al., 1972], OSO-7 (1971) [Thole, 1973] , HEAO-1 (1977) [Matteson, 1974] , RXTE (1995) [Gruber et al., 1996], BeppoSAX (1996) [Scarsi, 1997] , INTEGRAL (2002) [Hermsen and Winkler, 1998], Swift (2004) [Wells et al., 2004] and Astrosat-SSM (2015) [Seetha et al., 2006] used spatially coded mask technique for imaging X-ray sources.

X-ray imaging optics

At X-ray wavelength, most materials become transparent to photons as the refractive index of all materials is approximately equal to one. This makes normal incidence X-ray reflection optics very difficult. However, at very small angles from the surface, X-rays can be reflected which makes grazing incidence X-ray telescopes possible. Detailed discussion on X-ray mirrors and grazing incidence X-rays optics is included in Chapter 2. Wolter type I geometry [Wolter, 1952] is the most popular design for astronomical X-ray optics. Wolter type I optics consist of a parabolic profile primary mirror followed by a hyperbolic secondary mirror placed at very small angles to incident X-rays. X-ray optics not only enables the high spatial resolution X-ray imaging but also provides excellent signal to noise ratio observations due to to reduced background . X-ray detectors suffer from a large background component. The contribution of the background increases with the size of the detector. Hence without optics even by increasing the effective area of detectors, the signal to noise ratio is not improved substantially. Minimum detectable flux (S) of a collimated detector is given by 1.1

$$S = \frac{N}{\eta_E} \sqrt{\frac{2B}{A_d \Delta t \Delta E}} \tag{1.1}$$

where N is the confidence in observation, η_E is the quantum efficiency of the detector, B is background flux, A_d is the effective area of the detector, Δt is the integration time of the observation and ΔE the operational bandwidth of the detector. As A_d increases, correspondingly B also increases which keep the minimum detectable level high. But in case of a telescope with focusing optics, the total effective area of the instrument can be increased by increasing the size of optics by keeping the area of the detector very small. Minimum detectable flux S in-case of focussing optics is given by 1.2,

$$S = \frac{N}{A_o \eta_n} \sqrt{\frac{2BA_d}{\Delta t \Delta E}} \tag{1.2}$$

where A_o is the effective area of the optics which is typically several orders of magnitude higher than the area of the detector.

Several recent X-ray instruments use the high resolution, large effective area X-ray optics. A major challenge in X-ray optics lies in maintaining the balance between high-resolution imaging and large effective area. As mirrors are placed at very steep angles, the effective geometric area of the instrument is relatively very small. Hence a large number of concentric mirrors are placed in order to increase the effective area. A severe requirement in maintaining a large number of shells is to develop thin substrate mirrors. It is very difficult to maintain exact parabolic and hyperbolic profiles and figure errors on the mirror surface. This limits the spatial resolution of the instrument. Table 1.2 presents the details of several X-ray missions that are flown using X-ray optics.

Table 1.2: Details of several X-ray missions that are flown using X-ray optics.

Mission	Year	Focal length (m)	Area @ 1 keV (cm^2)	Upper energy (keV)	No. of shells	On-axis resolution
S-054/Skylab	1973	2.13	15	4	2	$48''$
S-056/Skylab	1973	1.90	9	1.3	1	$3''$
Einstein	1978	3.44	100	4	4	$4''$
EXOSAT	1983	1.09	70	2.5	2×2	$24''$
ROSAT	1990	2.4	420	2.5	4	$3''$
BBXRT	1990	3.77	450	12	2×118	$5''$
Yohkoh SXT	1991	1.54	23	4	1	$< 5''$
ASCA	1993	3.5	1200	10	4×120	$180''$
Soho CDS	1995	2.58	23	0.5	1	$< 5''$
BeppoSAX	1996	1.85	344	10	4×30	$60''$
ABRIXAS	1999	1.60	560	10	7×27	$25''$
Chandra	1999	10	780	10	4	$< 1''$
XMM-Newton	1999	7.5	4260	15	3×58	$16''$
Swift	2004	3.5	130	10	12	$18''$
Suzaku XRT-I	2005	4.70	450	12	4×175	$120''$
Suzaku XRT-S	2005	4.5	450	12	168	$120''$
NuSTAR	2012	10.15	800 @ 10 keV	79	133	$58''$
Astrosat-XST	2015	2	100	10	41	$120''$

X-ray telescopes are mainly limited with the narrow bandwidth (< 10 keV) and small effective area to weight ratio. The limitation is mainly due to the grazing incidence X-ray mirrors. Multilayer mirrors [Vinogradov and Zeldovich, 1977] working on the principle of Bragg's law can be a potential alternative to the conventional mirrors to develop broadband hard X-ray telescopes as well as large numerical aperture soft X-ray telescope. In the subsequent chapters, the design, fabrication, and characterization of multilayer mirrors is extensively discussed with some potential applications to the upcoming fields of X-ray astronomy.

1.4 Summary

In this chapter we have presented an overview of major science motivations in X-ray astronomy. We have also discussed all the techniques currently available for X-ray imaging, spectrometry and timing observations. In chapter 2 we will discuss in detail X-ray reflection optics by thin film mirrors and multilayer mirrors. Chapter 3 presents some of the fabrication and testing techniques of multilayer mirrors and also presents the experimental results from the fabricated W/B_4C multilayer mirrors. In chapter 4, we have presented the experimental results describing the performance stability of W/B_4C multilayer mirrors in the context of application to space-based instrumentation. Chapter 5 presents a novel design of multilayer mirror based soft X-ray polarimeter and a detailed discussion on the performance estimation and its relevance to observational X-ray astronomy. We have performed the deep Si etching on the non-reflecting side of multilayer mirror's substrate to increase the hard X-ray transmission efficiency of the mirror. These mirrors are useful for developing simultaneous instrument for soft and hard X-ray polarimetry using two detectors. These results are presented in chapter 6. Chapter 7 discusses a design concept of an X-ray instrument for planetary observations. This instrument consists of an X-ray concentrator to increase the signal to noise ratio of the observation. We have presented the summary of the thesis and future work in the final chapter 8.

Chapter 2

Thin film and multilayer X-ray mirrors

Instrumentation at X-ray wavelengths is mainly limited by the nature of the optical constants of materials. As the energy of photon in X-ray region is large compared to the binding energies of the electrons, optical properties of a material are mostly governed by the atomic scattering factors. Atomic scattering factor is a measure of scattering power of an isolated atom. If X-rays are scattered from an atom of atomic number 'Z', then the scattering amplitude is Z times the amplitude of a single electron, if all electrons scatter in the same direction. But not all electrons in an atom scatter in the same direction. Hence atomic scattering factor is defined as a ratio of the amplitude of the amplitude of wave scattered by an atom to the wave scattered by an electron. At large photon energies ($> 2keV$), the atomic scattering factor approaches the number of electrons per atom (i.e., the number of electrons with binding energies less than the photon energy). Hence the refractive index of different materials at X-ray region is distinguished only by the density of electrons.

Frequency (ω) dependent complex refractive index of the material with density

ρ is given by [Born and Wolf, 1975],

$$n(\omega) = 1 - \frac{\rho r_e \lambda^2}{2\pi}[f_1(\omega) - i f_2(\omega)] \qquad (2.1)$$

where, r_e is the classical radius of the electron, f_1 and f_2 are the wavelength dependent atomic scattering factors of the material. Imaginary part f_2 signifies the absorption or attenuation of the wave due to scattering. Equation (2.1) can also be written as,

$$n(\omega) = 1 - \delta + i\beta \qquad (2.2)$$

where,

$$\delta = \frac{r_e \rho \lambda^2}{2\pi} f_1(\omega) \qquad (2.3)$$

$$\beta = \frac{r_e \rho \lambda^2}{2\pi} f_2(\omega) \qquad (2.4)$$

2.1   X-ray reflection

The values of δ and β are extremely small at X-ray wavelengths and their values are very close for all elements. Table 2.1 shows the δ and β values of some elements at 2 keV. The real part of the refractive index is given by $1 - \delta$. Since δ is very small, the real part of the refractive index is very close to 1. The last column of table 2.1 gives the real part of the refractive index of respective materials.

From Fresnel equations, the normal incidence reflectivity of light travelling

Table 2.1: δ and β of various materials at 2 keV.

Material	δ	β	Re(n)
Tungsten	4.9×10^{-4}	3.5×10^{-4}	0.99951
Ruthenium	4.8×10^{-4}	6.7×10^{-5}	0.99952
Gold	5.2×10^{-4}	10.7×10^{-5}	0.99948
Aluminium	1.4×10^{-4}	3.0×10^{-5}	0.99986
Silicon	1.1×10^{-4}	3.1×10^{-5}	0.99989
Boron Carbide	1.3×10^{-4}	2.3×10^{-6}	0.99987

from medium with refractive index of n_1 to n_2 is given by,

$$R - \frac{n_2 - n_1}{n_2 + n_1} \qquad (2.5)$$

From table 2.1, it is observed that the real part of the refractive index is very close to one. Figure 2.1 shows the normal incidence reflectivity of different materials as a function of wavelength from 0.01 nm to 700 nm. The reflectivity drops very close to zero for all materials at shorter wavelengths. Hence X-ray reflectivity at normal incidence is negligible. However, X-ray reflection is possible when the angle of incidence is smaller than the critical angle for total external reflection. All angles are measured from the surface.

2.1.1 Critical angle for total external reflection

Reflection of x-rays from a surface is often termed as total external reflection instead of total internal reflection because the refractive index is usually less than one. The Critical angle is defined as the angle at which an incident ray is completely reflected. From Snell's law and figure 2.2 we have,

$$ncos(\theta_1) = (1 - \delta + i\beta)cos(\theta_r) \qquad (2.6)$$

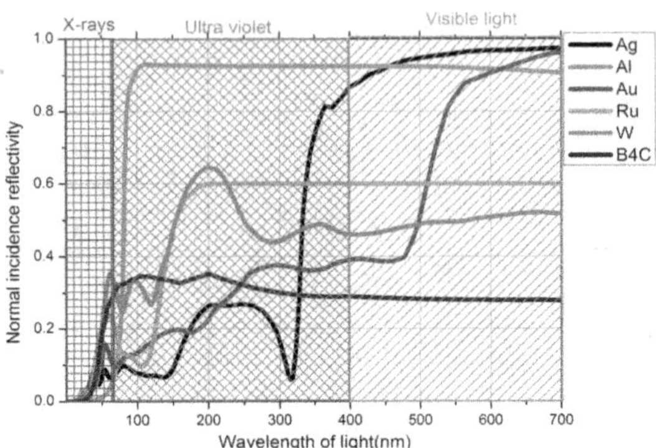

Figure 2.1: Normal incidence reflectivity of different materials as s function of wavelength of light from visible light to X-rays.

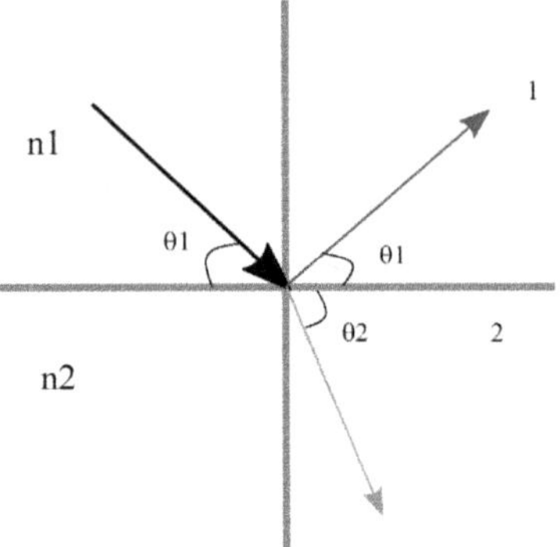

Figure 2.2: Reflection of X-rays at interface of two media.

If we neglect the contribution of the imaginary term 'β' and approximate $n = 1$ then equation (2.6) reduces to,

$$cos(\theta_1) = (1 - \delta)cos(\theta_r) \qquad (2.7)$$

Total external reflection occurs when a refracted wave is completely absent. i.e.

equation (2.7) has no solution for θ_r. Since the angle at which θ_r has no solution, it is called the critical angle, θ_1 is substituted as θ_c. Deriving for θ_c we get,

$$\cos(\theta_r) = \frac{\cos(\theta_c)}{(1 - \delta)} \geq 1 \tag{2.8}$$

$$\cos(\theta_c) = (1 - \delta) \tag{2.9}$$

Approximating $cos(\theta_c)$ at small angles,

$$1 - \frac{\theta_c^2}{2} = 1 - \delta \tag{2.10}$$

$$\theta_c = \sqrt{2\delta} \tag{2.11}$$

But we know form equation (2.3) that, δ is a function of ρ & λ^2. Hence,

$$\delta \propto \lambda^2 \rho$$

$$\theta_c \propto \sqrt{\rho}\lambda$$

$$\theta_c \propto \frac{\sqrt{\rho}}{E} \tag{2.12}$$

Empirically, θ_c is observed [Bass et al., 2010],

$$\boldsymbol{\theta_c = 69' \frac{\sqrt{\rho}}{E}} \tag{2.13}$$

Here 'E' is the energy of the incident photon in keV. Figure 2.3 shows the calculated reflectivity curve as a function of incident angle at different energies for a tungsten mirror.

From figure 2.3, it is observed that the X-ray reflectivity is confined to very

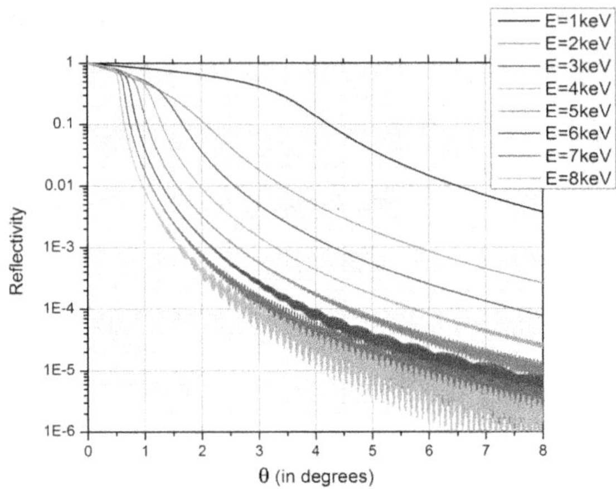

Figure 2.3: Reflectivity of a tungsten (W) coated x-ray mirror for different incident photon energies as a function of incident angle. As energy of input x-rays increases, critical angle decreases. These plots are obtained by modeling the mirror using IMD software [Windt, 1998].

small angles below the critical angle. As the energy of incident X-rays increases, the critical angle decreases and hence reflectivity is restricted to small angles. Reflectivity is close to 1 for very small angles. In total reflection regime the reflection takes place at very small depths, thus the photoelectric absorption is negligible. Reflectivity for a given angle is directly proportional to δ of reflecting material to produce the contrast for reflection and inversely proportional to β to minimize the absorption. For small incidence angles, the reflection efficiency can be approximated as,

$$R(\theta \ll \theta_c) \simeq 1 - 2\theta_{radians}\frac{\beta}{\delta^{\frac{3}{2}}} \tag{2.14}$$

Equation (2.14) is valid only when incidence angle is smaller than the critical angle and $\beta/\delta \ll 1$.

2.2 Grazing incidence X-ray reflection

2.2.1 Thickness of the thin film

From equation (2.12) it is evident that the high density reflecting surfaces have a large critical angle and also large bandpass of reflection. Hence grazing incidence (small angle from the surface) X-ray mirrors consists of a thin metallic film coated on a smooth substrate. The thickness of the metallic film is usually the order of a few tens of nanometers. The minimum thickness of the metallic layer for total external reflection depends on the energy of incident photons, the angle of incidence and the density of the metal. The critical thickness of the metallic layer at a given energy is defined as a minimum thickness of the thin film required for total external reflection of X-rays. X-ray reflectivity saturates over this thickness limit. Figure 2.4 shows the simulated reflectivity of gold (Au) coated mirror at 0.4^o as a function of the thickness of the Au layer for different energies. For small layer thickness mirrors, the reflectivity is very low as X-rays penetrate through the mirror material with minimal interaction. As the thickness increases, the reflectivity saturates to a critical value for total external reflection. Saturated reflectivity is less than unity due to absorption of X-ray in the reflecting medium. It is observed that, as the energy of incident photon increases, the saturation value of thickness increases. This is due to an increase in penetration depth with photon energy.

2.2.2 Keissig oscillations

The thickness of the thin film also affects the reflectivity profile of the mirror at higher angles (above critical angles). Above critical angle, most of the X-rays get penetrated into the reflecting material with very little reflection from the top surface. Since reflecting layer is coated on a solid substrate, the pene-

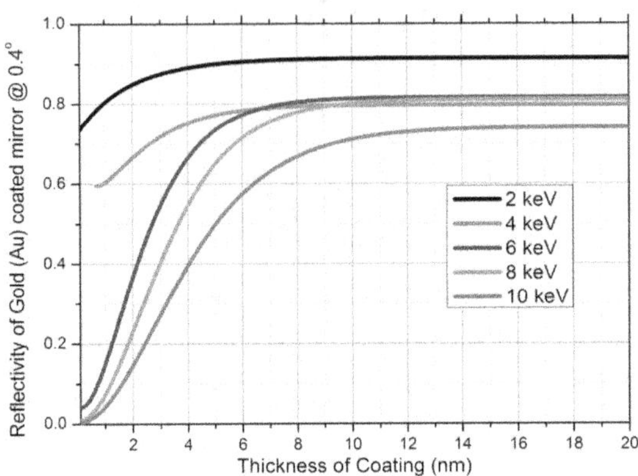

Figure 2.4: Reflectivity of gold (Au) coated mirror at 0.4^o (less than critical angle) as a function of thickness of Au layer for different photon energy. Reflectivity saturates as the thickness increases and saturation value is higher for high energy X-rays.

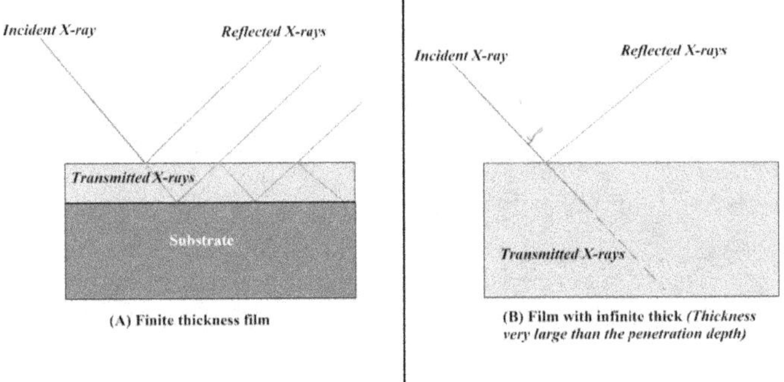

Figure 2.5: Schematic representing effect of thickness of metallic layer on multiple reflections. Part A shown the case of finite thickness layer where multiple reflections are formed due to partial reflection from the interfaces. Part B on the right is for a case of large thickness layer where multiple reflections do not occur.

trated X-rays also gets partially reflected from the thin film- substrate interface. Reflected X-rays from the substrate again gets partially reflected and transmitted

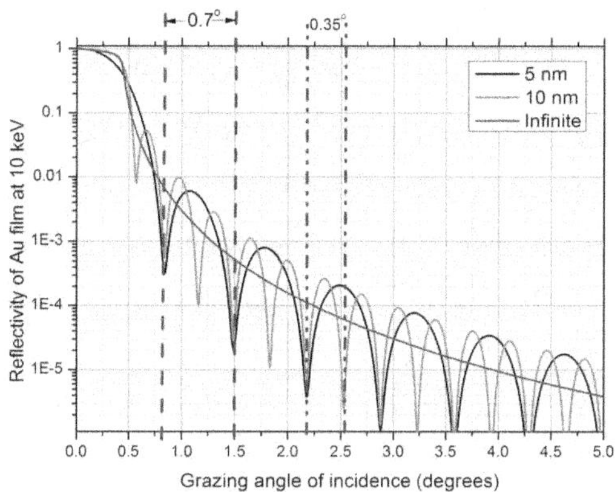

Figure 2.6: Reflectivity of gold (Au) coated mirror as a function of incident angles for mirrors with different thickness. Keissig oscillations are formed above critical for finite thickness Au layer mirrors. Period of oscillation reduces as the thickness of the reflecting layer increases.

from the thin film-ambient interface. For a monochromatic X-ray source, all the partially reflected rays will constructively interfere periodically for certain angles of incidence. These form oscillation in the reflectivity curve know as Keissig oscillations [Nigam, 1965]. Period of Keissig oscillation depends on the thickness of the metallic layer. Though these oscillation cause very low reflectivity patterns, these are used ex-situ measurements of the thickness of the thin film. As the thickness of the reflecting layer increases, the period of Keissig oscillation reduces. Figure 2.5 shows the schematic of an X-ray mirror producing multiple internal reflections above the critical angle. Part (b) of the shown a case where the thickness of the reflecting surface is very large (larger than the penetration depth). In this case, Keissig oscillation does not occur as there are no multiple reflections. Figure 2.6 shows the simulated reflectivity profile of Au mirrors of different thickness on a Si substrate as a function of incident angle at 10 keV. Three profiles correspond to mirrors with three different thickness of the Au layer as given in the inset.

For the mirror with infinite thickness (larger than the penetration depth), the reflectivity smoothly drops exponentially in log scale above the critical angle. But in the case of finite thickness mirrors (10 nm and 5 nm), Keissig oscillations are observed. These oscillations have very low reflectivity and decay very rapidly for higher order oscillations. The period of oscillations is a function of the thickness of the reflecting layer and the energy of the incident photon. From the figure, it is observed that the period of oscillation of 5 nm thick Au mirror is 0.7^o and as the thickness doubles to 10 nm, the period of oscillation becomes half to 0.35^o.

Since the Keissig oscillations are formed by the multiple reflections from the thin film and the substrate, the contrast in densities of thin film and the substrate governs the contrast of oscillations. A small difference in the densities results in less contrast of oscillations. Figure 2.7 shows IMD simulated reflectivity profiles of Au coated mirror as a function of incident angle at 10 keV with two different substrates. The difference in the densities of Nickel (Ni) (8.9 g/cc) and Au (18.3 g/cc) is lower than Silicon (Si) (2.2 g/cc) and Au. Hence the contrast of Keissig oscillations with Si substrate is higher than with Ni substrate.

2.2.3 Surface micro-roughness

Grazing incidence X-ray reflectivity is greatly affected by the micro-roughness of the reflecting surface. The mirror surface has to be smooth in order to attain a reflectivity near to the value predicted by Fresnel laws. Several super polishing techniques are being developed to reduce the RMS roughness from micrometer to sub-nanometer scale. However, a real mirror will always have a non-zero roughness which reduces the reflectivity.Equation (2.14) gives the grazing angle X-ray reflectivity of a smooth surface. Effects of micro-roughness on reflectivity are also energy and angle of incidence dependent. Reflectivity from a rough surface R_σ

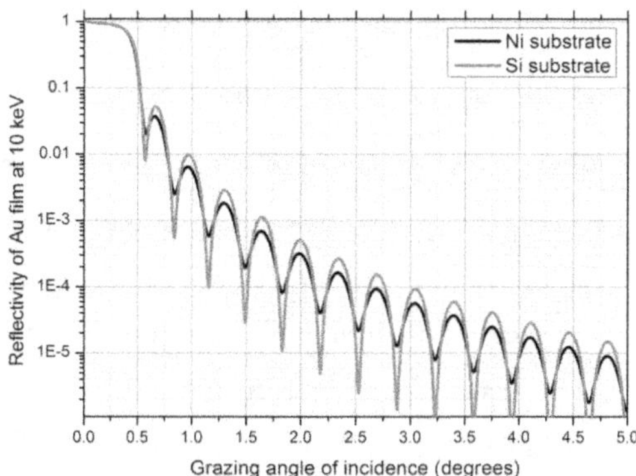

Figure 2.7: Reflectivity of gold (Au) coated mirror as a function of incident angles with two different substrates (Ni and Si). The contrast of Keissig oscillations is higher with Si substrate than with Ni substrate as the difference between the densities of Au and Si is higher than the difference between Au and Ni.

with RMS roughness σ given by (2.15):

$$R_\sigma(\theta) = R(\theta).(1 - Q) \qquad (2.15)$$

where the value of Q depends on the spatial correlation length (ξ) of the roughness. Spatial correlation length of a surface is the defined as the length scales at which roughness amplitude is of the order of wavelength of light. If the spatial correlation length of roughness is very high ($\xi \to \infty$), then Q is given by $Debye - Waller$ (DW) relation (5.30). When the roughness correlation length is close to zero ($\xi \to 0$), then the value of Q is given by $Nevot - Croce$ (NC) relation (2.17) [Spiller, 1996].

$$Q_{DW} = \left(\frac{4\pi\sigma \sin\theta}{\lambda}\right)^2 . \forall \xi \to \infty \qquad (2.16)$$

$$Q_{NC} = \left(\frac{4\,pi\sigma}{\lambda}\right)^2 . \sin\theta\, Re\,\sqrt{\xi - \cos^2\theta} . \forall \xi \to 0 \qquad (2.17)$$

From (2.15), (5.30) and (2.17), one can infer that the effect of micro-roughness is larger for a larger angle on incidence and for the small wavelength of the incident photon. Figure 2.8 shows the simulated reflectivity profiles of Au coated mirror at 0.5^o as a function of incident photon energy for the different roughness of the mirror. As the roughness increases, the grazing incidence reflectivity reduces. And the effect is higher for higher energies. A sudden drop of reflectivity near 2 keV is due to the absorption edge of gold (Au).

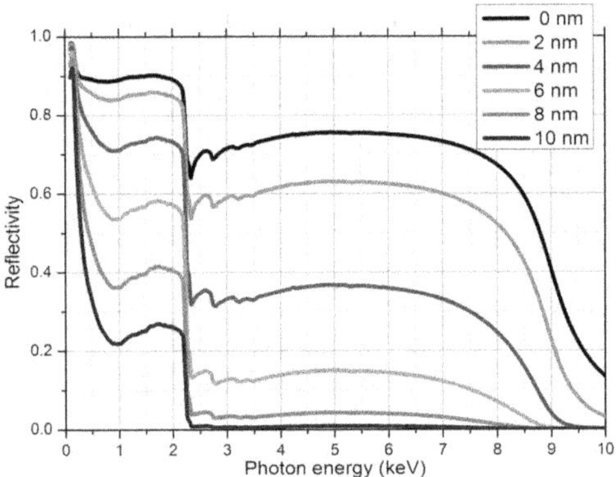

Figure 2.8: Simulated reflectivity profiles of a Au coated mirror at 0.5^o as a function of photon energy for different RMS roughness of the mirror. RMS roughness in nanometers (nm) in given in the inset.

2.3   X-ray transmission from thin films

As the refractive index of all mediums is nearly equal to 1 at X-ray wavelength, rays transmit through all the materials when incident well above critical angle (eq. (2.13)). However, X-rays are absorbed by the medium by inelastic scattering of an electron in the material. X-ray absorption exponentially increases with the increase in the density of the material. The imaginary term the complex refractive index β (eq.(2.4)) gives the absorption component of X-rays in a medium. As the thickness of film increases, the transmission efficiency reduces due to increase in absorption. Figure 2.9 show the transmission efficiency of different material films at 8 keV as a function of the thickness of the film. From the figure, it is evident that fewer density materials like Si and Al have high transmission efficiency even with a large thickness. This is due to less absorption of X-rays from low dens material. X-ray transmission filters are often used high pass filters as transmission efficiency of a given filter increases as the incident photon energy increases.

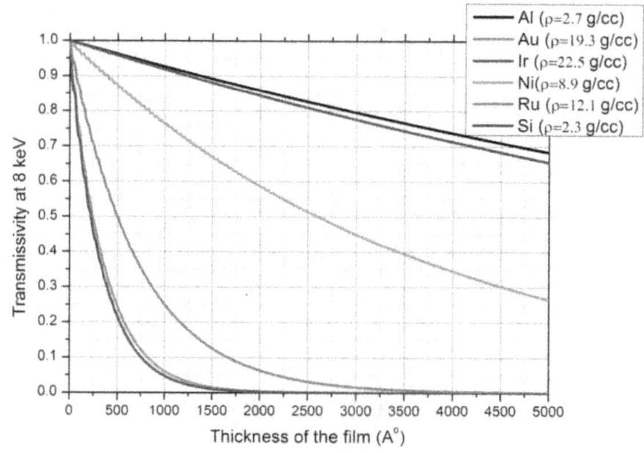

Figure 2.9: Normal incidence transmission efficiency of various materials at 8 keV as a function of the thickness. High density materials have less transmission efficiency due to high absorption.

2.4 X-ray filters

For a mirror of a given material, the critical angle of X-ray reflection reduces with the energy of the incident photon. Hence at a given angle of incidence, the reflectivity of X-rays rapidly falls above a certain energy. Hence grazing incidence X-ray reflection mirrors act as low pass filter whose passband depends on the incident angle and the density of the material. X-ray transmission filters act a natural high pass filter which attenuates low energy X-rays. Hence in a combination of both reflecting mirrors and transmission filters, one can design a moderate resolution notch filter with a very narrow passband. Figure 2.10 shows the design of two moderate resolution notch filters with different materials and configurations. In an example given in figure 2.10 a 4 keV notch filter is designed by a Ni X-ray mirror at 0.83^o which is close to the critical angle of Ni at 4 keV. And a Ni filter with thickness 7.5 μm is used as a filter which absorbs all the low energy X-rays. When the response of both the filter and mirror are convolved, we get a narrow passband at 4 keV. Similarly, a gold mirror at 1.5^o with a 5 μm Yttrium acts as a notch filter at 2 keV. The sharp cut-off just above 2 keV is due to the absorption edge of Yttrium at 2.1 keV. Similarly one can design notch filter for other bands by properly design mirror and filter configurations.

2.5 Grazing incidence X-ray optics

A truncated parabolic shell acts as a grazing incidence X-ray focusing optical system with large focal length (small angle of incidence). However, the parabolic shape cannot be used as an imaging telescope as it is affected by strong 'coma' aberration for off-axis sources. As a result, the active imaging field of view is very small for a parabolic reflector. A coma-free optic can be developed if the Abbe

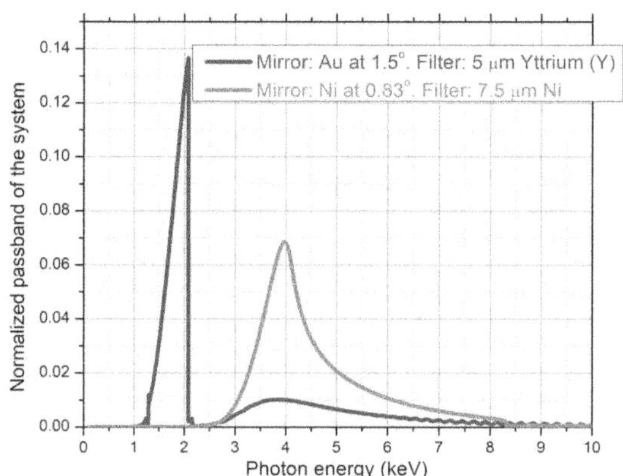

Figure 2.10: Moderate resolution notch filter 2 keV and 4 keV designed in combination of X-ray mirror and transmission filter.

sine condition [gM.A., 1910] (2.18) is satisfied in all points of the reflecting surface.

$$\frac{h}{\sin \alpha_i} = \frac{i}{\sin \alpha_o} = constant \tag{2.18}$$

where h and i denote the distance of the object and image point from the optical axis respectively. α_i, α_o are the angle between the ray after reflection and the optical axis respectively. The Abbe condition rules out a single parabolic reflector for coma-free off-axis imaging.

A solution to this problem is given by Hans Wolter in 1951 [Wolter, 1952] where he showed that the Abbe condition could be approximately satisfied by using a double reflection on two conical mirrors in succession. Double reflection also reduces the focal length of optics by a factor of 2. Wolter came with three different configurations which suppress off-axis coma by double reflection. Figure 2.11 shows the optical schematic of Wolter type I, II, and III designs. Among them, Wolter type I design is very popular among astronomical X-ray telescopes as it has the shortest focal length for the same aperture when compared to type II and types III designs.

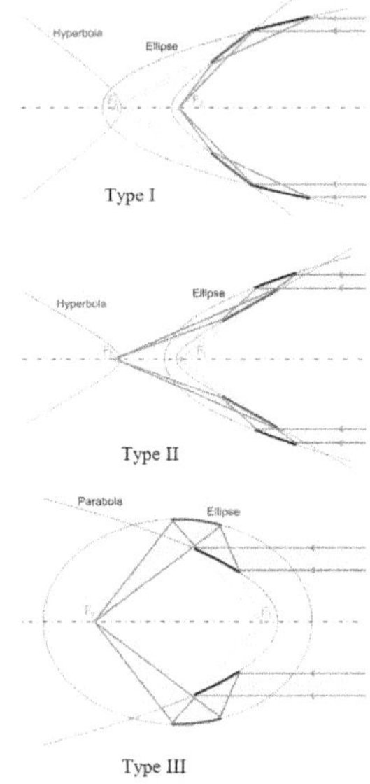

Figure 2.11: Optical schematics of Wolter type I (top), type II (middle) and type III (bottom) designs with double reflection to eliminate coma aberration for off-axis imaging. Picture credit: $http://www.x-ray-optics.de/index.php/en/types-of-optics/reflecting-optics/curved-mirrors$

An X-ray telescope with Wolter type I optics has a circular radial profile and parabolic and hyperbolic axial profiles for primary and secondary mirrors respectively. Since these mirrors are operated at very small angles of incidence, the effective geometric area of the telescope is very small when compared to the physical geometric area of the instrument. Secondary hyperbolic profile mirror will not contribute to increasing the overall effective area of the telescope but it is used to reduce the focal length and enhance the imaging properties. Energy-dependent effective area of Wolter type I optics is given by (2.19):

$$A_e(E) = 2\pi r l \sin\theta R_1(E).R_2(E) \qquad (2.19)$$

where l is the axial length of the primary mirror, r is the radius of the primary mirror, θ is the inclination angle of the primary mirror with respect optical axis, $R_1(E)$ and $R_2(E)$ and the energy-dependent X-ray reflectivities of the primary and secondary mirrors. In order to get 100% throughput, the primary and secondary mirrors should satisfy the condition (2.20)

$$l_1 \sin\theta_1 = l_2 \sin\theta_2 \qquad (2.20)$$

where l_1, l_2 are the axial lengths of primary and secondary mirrors respectively. θ_1 and θ_2 are the inclination of the primary mirror with respect to the optical axis and the inclination of the secondary mirror with respect to the primary mirror respectively. Equation (2.20) gives the condition for all on-axis rays reflected from the primary mirror to be reflected from the secondary mirror without any loss. In most practical cases, l_1 and l_2 are kept equal and hence θ_1 and θ_2 are also equal. If similar reflective coating is applied to the primary and secondary mirrors, the $R_1(E) = R_2(E) = R(E)$. These conditions converges (2.19) to:

$$A_e(E) = 2\pi r l \sin\theta R^2(E) \qquad (2.21)$$

Focal length (f) of Wolter type I optics depends on the radius of the primary mirror and the angle of incidence which is given by (2.22):

$$\frac{r}{f} = tan(4\theta) \qquad (2.22)$$

4θ is the convergence angle of the beam after double reflection as each reflection adds the convergence angle of 2θ. Since the effective area of Wolter type I design is very small for small incidence angles, astronomical X-ray telescopes adopt the technique of concentric shells design. In this design, several primary and secondary shells are placed concentric to each. Angles of incidence of concentric shells are varied according to the radius of the shell to have a common focal length of all shells as per (2.22). To maximize the packing density for concentric shells, the thickness of the mirror should be reduced. Several advanced fabrication techniques are being employed to develop thin X-rays mirrors to enhance the packing density of the telescope. Chandra X-ray telescope mirror is 20 mm thick [Zombeck et al., 1981] while XMM-Newton mirrors 1 mm thick [Koch-Miramond, 1985]. Recent X-ray telescopes like SXT- Astrosat developed 0.5 mm thick mirrors by replication technique [Singh et al., 2017a]. Spektr-RG X-ray telescope developed 0.25 mm thick mirrors [Arefiev et al., 2008] and future instruments like MiXO are developing 0.2 mm thick X-ray mirrors [Hong et al., 2014] by more advanced techniques.

While thin foil X-ray mirrors are used to increase the packing density and effective area per mass ration of the telescope, it is very difficult to produce and maintains parabolic and hyperbolic axial profiles on the mirrors. This will greatly affect the imaging quality of an X-ray telescope. Chandra X-ray telescope used properly figured thick glass substrates which maintained parabolic and hyperbolic profiles while the contemporary XMM- Newton used electroformed Ni substrate with a conical approximation. As a result, the angular resolution of Chandra X-ray telescope is 0.5 arc second and that of XMM-Newton is 6 arc second [Dubner et al., 2017]. Figure 2.12 shows the comparison of the image of Crab nebula recorded from Chandra and XMM- Newton X-ray telescopes. From the figure 2.12, one can clearly see the jets from crab pulsar and structure around it from Chandra image which is not very clear from the XMM- Newton image. On the other hand effective area per mass ratio of Chandra is just 0.54 cm^2/kg while it is 4.34 cm^2/kg

for XMM- Newton telescope.

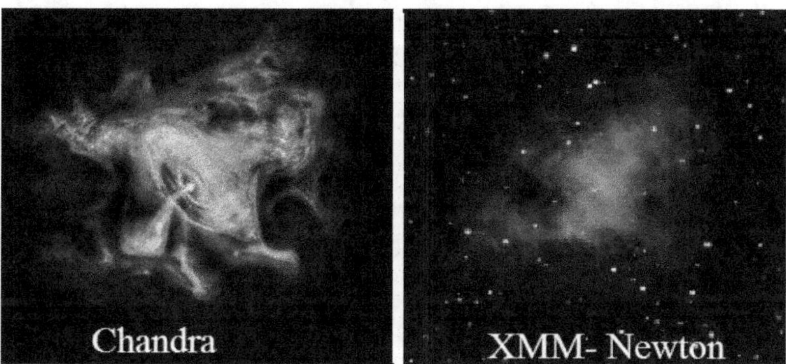

Figure 2.12: Comparison of image of Crab nebula recorded from Chandra (left) and XMM- Newton (right) X-ray telescopes. Reference" [Dubner et al., 2017]

2.5.1   X-ray concentrators

Wolter type I design is used for high-resolution X-ray imaging and for moderate resolution imaging, a conical approximation of Wolter type I design is used for Astronomical X-ray telescopes. Imaging telescopes are heavy, expensive and difficult to align and calibrate. But if the aim of the instrument is just to concentrate more X-rays on a small detector with high signal to noise ratio and not to image, a simple single reflection optics can still be useful. Such systems are less expensive, easy to align and have less weight. For applications such as not imaging photon counting, spectroscopy, and polarimetry, a simple X-ray concentrator is used to increase the signal to noise ratio. However, the concentrators have larger focal length which increases the overall size of the instrument. Since they have a single reflector, their effective area is given by (2.23):

$$A_e(e) = 2\pi r l \sin\theta R(E) \tag{2.23}$$

and the relation between radius and focal length for given angle of incidence is given by (2.24):

$$\frac{r}{f} = tan(2\theta) \tag{2.24}$$

For a concentrator with 'n' number of concentric shells, the outer radius of $n-1^{th}$ shell should not occult the inner radius of nth shell. And angle incidence of all shells should vary according to (2.24) with the respective radius of the shell to have a common focus. This leads to a set of conditions which needs to be satisfied for 100% throughput concentrator. This should also consider the thickness of the clearance mirror and the gap left between two concentric shells for mechanical and field of view considerations.

Let r_n^1, r_n^2 and θ_n be the outer and inner radii and angle of incidence of the 'n^{th}' shell respectively. Let 'l' be the length of each shell, 'g' be gap between two shells, 't' the thickness of the mirror substrate and 'f' the focal length of the mirror. From figure 2.13,

$$r_1^2 = r_1^1 - l \sin \theta_1 \tag{2.25}$$

Considering radius of each shell from the center of the shell i.e. $\frac{r_n^1 + r_n^2}{2}$,

$$\frac{r_1^1 + r_1^2}{2f} = \sin 2\theta \tag{2.26}$$

By solving equations (2.25) and (2.26) for θ, we get,

$$2f \sin 2\theta + l \sin \theta - 2r_1^1 = 0 \tag{2.27}$$

Since f,l and r_1^1 are known to begin with, we can solve equation (2.27) to find out angle of incidence of first shell 'θ_1' and hence from equation (2.25), r_1^2 can be calculated.

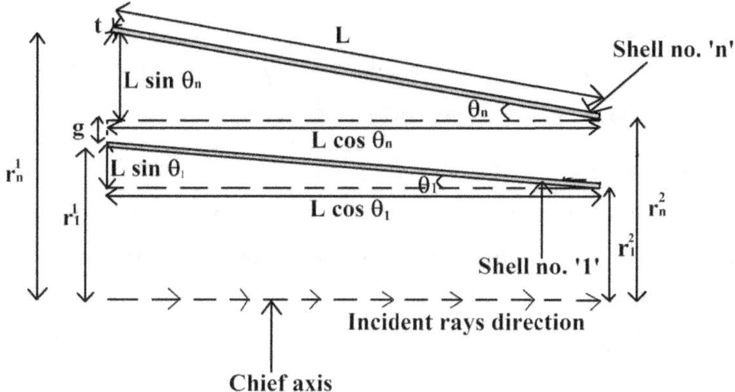

Figure 2.13: Schematic of concentric placement for no vignetting condition in case of single reflection X-ray concentrator.

Calculation of shell's specification for n^{th} shell Specifications of nth shell depends on the specifications of $(n-1)^{th}$ shell. Inner radius of nth shell without any vignetting effect is given by,

$$r_n^2 = r_{n-1}^1 + g + t \tag{2.28}$$

From figure 2.13 and equation (2.24), we get following equations respectively,

$$r_n^1 = r_n^2 + l \sin \theta_n \tag{2.29}$$

$$\frac{r_n^1 + r_n^2}{2f} = \sin 2\theta_n \tag{2.30}$$

Solving equations (2.29) and (2.30) for θ, we get,

$$2f \sin 2\theta_n - l \sin \theta_n - 2r_n^2 = 0 \tag{2.31}$$

From above equations, one can calculate r_n^1, r_n^2 and θ_n for 'n' number of shells for a single reflection conic approximated concentrators.

Several alternative designs like Montel-optics, Kirkpatrick-Baez (KB) optics, cylindrical Wolter optics, polycapillary optics, Si pore optics etc. uses the principle of grazing incidence X-ray optics to focus X-rays for various applications.

2.6 Multilayer mirrors

Major limitations of optics developed with grazing incidence mirror are its low effective area and large focal length. These limitations are primarily due to the small critical angle for total external reflection. This also limits the high energy cut-off of X-ray telescopes typically under 10 keV. Optics developed with small angle reflection mirror also limits the active field of view of the X-ray telescope. Multilayer coating mirrors or simply 'multilayer mirrors' provide a solution to these limitations by reflecting soft X-rays at large angles for a large effective area and short focal length optics and also reflecting hard X-rays (~ 100 keV) for large bandwidth X-ray telescopes [Christensen et al., 1995], [Krieger et al., 1997], [Mao et al., 1997], [Tawara et al., 1998]. Multilayer mirrors can also be used for normal incidence EUV- soft X-ray mirrors [Evans et al., 1989], [Evans et al., 1988], [Windt et al., 2004] as well as for soft X-ray polarimeters [Marshall et al., 1998], [Grimmer et al., 2001], [Marshall et al., 2010], [Marshall et al., 2014], [Marshall, 2015], [She et al., 2015], [Panini et al., 2018].

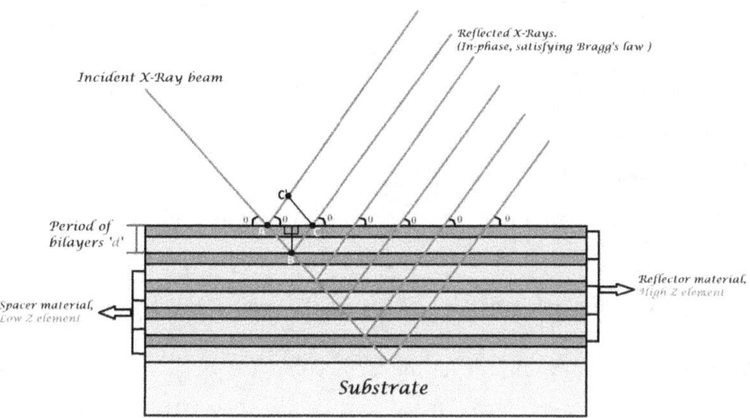

Figure 2.14: A schematic representing the working principle of multilayer mirrors for X-rays above critical angle of total reflection.

Multilayer mirrors consist of thin, periodic repetitive coatings of low- and high-density (or atomic number (Z)) materials with sharp interfaces as shown in figure 2.14. Multilayer mirrors work on the principle of constructive interference from thin layers of materials. When X-rays are incident at angles larger than the critical angle, most of the X-rays get transmitted through the top layer with a very low reflectivity. Since there is a sequence of contrasting layers, the transmitted X-rays get divided into transmitted and partially reflected component as each layer interface. The coating thickness of each layer can be optimized to interfere constructively all reflected component from all layers enhancing the overall reflectivity. However, as X-rays pass through layer material, a significant component of it will be absorbed in the media. Higher the density of the material, higher the absorption. Hence a single layer is subdivided into a high-density layer (reflector) and a low-density layer (spacer). While X-rays efficiently gets reflected from the reflector layer, the spacer layer helps in reducing the absorption of X-rays while passing through it. Contrasting densities of reflector and spacer layers not only minimize the absorption of X-rays but also provides excellent contrast for maximizing the reflectivity from each layer. A single layer consisting a reflector and a spacer layer is called a bilayer. Bilayers are repeated with periodicity' which is physically the thickness of one reflector layer and a spacer layer together.

2.6.1 Working principle of multilayer mirrors

X-ray reflectivity from a multilayer mirror is enhanced when the reflected component from all the reflector layers is constructively added. For constructive interference of X-rays, the effective path-length traveled by X-ray from all reflecting layers should be equal to the integral multiples of the wavelength. If an X-ray beam of wavelength λ is incident on a multilayer mirror at an angle θ $(> \theta_c)$, the additional path length traveled by the ray into the mirror should be equal to an integral multiple of λ. From figure 2.14,

$$
\begin{aligned}
n\lambda &= AB + BC - AC' \qquad (2.32)\\
&= \frac{d}{\sin\theta} + \frac{d}{\sin\theta} - AC\cos\theta\\
&= \frac{2d}{\sin\theta} - \frac{2d\cos\theta}{\tan\theta}\\
&= \frac{2d}{\sin\theta} - \frac{2d\cos^2\theta}{\sin\theta}\\
&= \frac{2d}{\sin\theta}(1 - \cos^2\theta)
\end{aligned}
$$

$$
\boldsymbol{n\lambda = 2d\sin\theta} \qquad (2.33)
$$

Equation (2.33) is called Bragg's law which gives the condition for reflection of X-rays from a multilayer mirror at angles above the critical angle. From the nature of equation (2.33), enhanced reflectivity is obtained only for narrow bands whenever the condition is satisfied for integer 'n'. These narrowband peaks of reflectivity are called Bragg peaks whose intensity rapidly falls as the 'n' (order of Bragg peak) increases. Figure 2.15 and 2.16 shows the typical reflectivity profiles of multilayer mirrors as a function of the angle of incidence for a monochromatic source and for different photon energies at a fixed angle respectively. These profiles are simulated using IMD software [Windt, 1998].

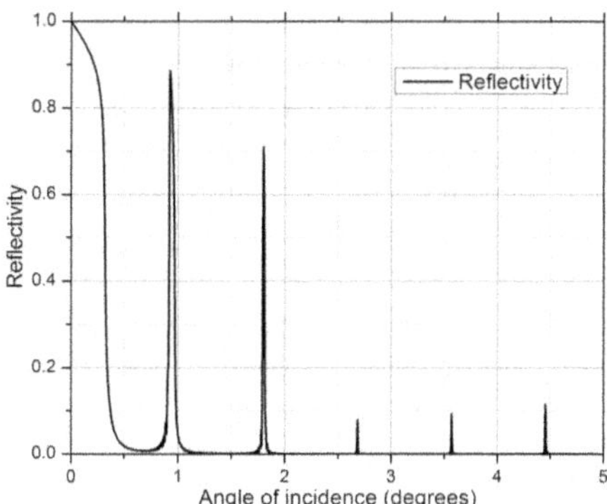

Figure 2.15: Calculated X-ray reflectivity profile at 8 keV as a function of incident angle for a modelled multilayer mirror with Ruthenium reflector and B_4C spacer layers with period of 5 nm.

In order to calculate the structure-function of a multilayer mirror, each layer pair of thickness d is considered as a unit cell. The angle-dependent structure-function along the direction normal to the mirror surface x of a unit cell is given by (2.34) [Michette, 1986]

$$F(\theta) = \int_0^d \phi(x) exp[4\pi i(\sin\theta)x/\lambda]dx \qquad (2.34)$$

where ϕ is the scattering amplitude density which depends on the material

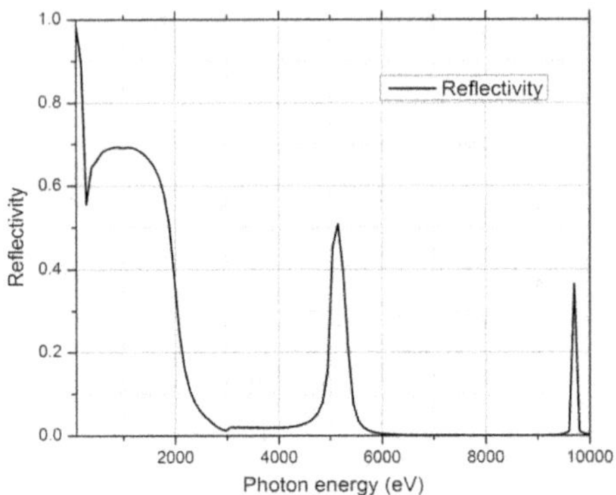

Figure 2.16: Calculated X-ray reflectivity profile as a function of different incident energies for modelled Ru-B_4C MCM with period of 5nm at 1.5^o.

properties as is given by (2.35) [Michette, 1986]:

$$\phi = \rho[(Z + \delta f_1^2) + f_2^2]^{1/2}e^2/4\pi\varepsilon_o m_e c^2 \qquad (2.35)$$

where ρ is the number density of atoms, c is the velocity of light and ϵ is the relative permittivity of the medium. If both reflector and spacer layers are homogeneous with scattering amplitudes ϕ_r and ϕ_s respectively and the interfaces are perfectively sharp, then the equation (2.34) can be written as (2.36):

$$F(\theta) = \int_0^{d_r} \phi_r exp(iQx)dx + \int_o^{d_s} \phi_s exp(iQx)dx \qquad (2.36)$$

where Q is momentum transfer a interface which is given by (2.37):

$$Q = \frac{4\pi \sin\theta}{\lambda} \qquad (2.37)$$

by solving the integrals of equation (2.36), we get (2.38):

$$F(\theta) = (1/iQ)[(\phi_s - \phi_r)expiQd_s - \phi_s + \phi_r expiQd] \qquad (2.38)$$

Magnitude of the above equation is given by (2.39)

$$|F(\theta)| = \frac{\sqrt{2}}{Q}[\phi_s^2(1-\cos Qd_s)+\phi_r^2(1-\cos Qd_r)-\phi_s\phi_r(1+\cos Qd-\cos Qd_s-\cos Qd_r)]$$

$$(2.39)$$

Let γ be the ratio of thickness of reflector material (d_r) to the period of bilayer (d). Then $d_r = \gamma d$ and $d_s = d - \gamma d$. Substituting d_r and d_s in terms of γ in equation (2.39), we get (2.40)

$$|F(\theta)| = \frac{\sqrt{2}}{Q}[\phi_s^2(1-\cos(Q(d-\gamma d)))+\phi_r^2(1-\cos Q\gamma d)-\phi_s\phi_r(1+\cos Qd-\cos(Q(d-\gamma d))-\cos Q\gamma d)]$$

$$(2.40)$$

At Bragg peaks, substituting $\sin\theta/\lambda = n\,2\pi$ in equation (2.37) we get,$Q = 2n\pi/d$ and $\cos Qd = 1$. Equation (2.40) gives the angle dependent structure function of a single unit cell (one bilayer) with sharp layer interface.

Neglecting the X-ray absorption from multilayers, the overall intensity of the reflected beam is estimated by Ewald solution which considers overall effect due to N number of bilayers in multilayer mirror. If X-rays of intensity I_o are incident on a multilayer mirror, then the angle-dependent reflected intensity ($I(\theta)$) is given by (2.41):

$$I(\theta) = I_o|p^2 + (p^2 - 1)\cot^2[A(p^2 - 1)^{0.5}]|^{-1} \tag{2.41}$$

where

$$A = (2Nkd/n)|F(\theta)| \tag{2.42}$$

$$p = (\pi n N/2A\sin^2\theta_n)[(\theta - \theta_n)\sin 2\theta_n - 2\delta] \tag{2.43}$$

the value of k depends on the state of polarization of incident X-rays which is given by

$$k = 1, \qquad\qquad Parallel$$
$$= |\cos 2\theta_m|, \qquad\qquad Perpendicular \qquad\qquad (2.44)$$
$$= (1 + |\cos 2\theta_m|)/2 \qquad unpolarized$$

when angle of incidence is equal to Bragg angle (i.e. $\theta = \theta_n$), reflectivity is maximized. Multilayer mirrors are considered thick if $A > 1.8$ and thin if $A < 0.4$.

Multilayer mirrors as polarizing elements: As the value of K depends on the polarization state of the incident photon, the response of multilayer mirrors varies according to the polarization of X-rays. For small as well as near normal incident angles, K for parallel and perpendicular polarization states are nearly equal. However when the angle of incidence is close to 45°, $k = \cos 2\theta$ becomes zero for perpendicular polarization state which completely suppresses the reflected component. When unpolarized X-rays are incident to a multilayer mirror with Bragg peak at 45°, only parallel component of X-rays are reflected. X-ray reflection at 45° satisfies Brewster's law [Brewster, 1815] which acts as a reflecting polarization element. Figure 2.17 shows the simulated reflectivity profile of a Co-C multilayer mirror with d= 3.5 nm at 45° as a function of incident photon energy for S- (parallel) and P- (perpendicular) polarization states of incident photons. S- polarization reflectivity of the mirror is more than 3 order of magnitude higher than the P-polarization reflectivity at 45°. This property of multilayer mirrors is exploited in developing soft X-ray polarimeters. More on soft X-ray polarimeters is discussed in Chapter 6.

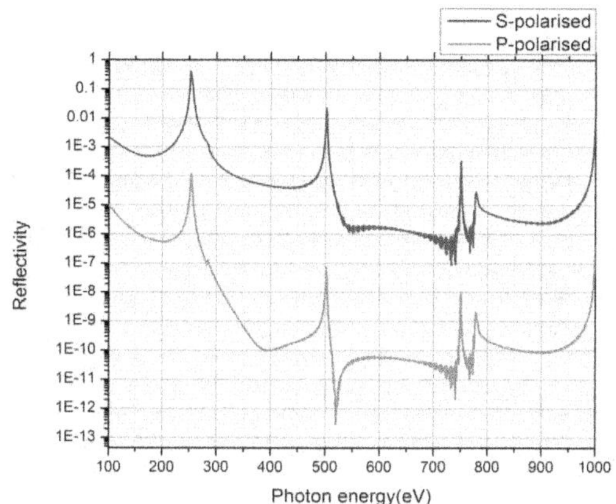

Figure 2.17: Reflectivity profile of a Co-C multilayer mirror at 45° as a function of incidence photon energy for S- (parallel) and P- (perpendicular) polarization states.

2.6.2   Effect of number of bilayers

From equations (2.41) and (2.42), it is evident that as A increases, reflectivity increases. A is directly proportional to the number of bilayers N, Reflectivity at Bragg peaks can be enhanced by fabricating a multilayer mirror with a large number of bilayers. If the medium is non-absorbing, ideally it is possible to develop mirrors with 100% reflectivity for large N. However, X-rays get absorbed by thin films in multilayer mirrors. This gives a limit on a total number of effective number of bilayers (N_{eff}) which is given by (2.45) [Michette, 1986]:

$$N_{eff} = n^2 \pi A / [2kd^2(\phi_r - \phi_s)\sin(m\pi d_r/d)] \tag{2.45}$$

From the nature of equation (2.45), it is noted that N_{eff} is a function period of the bilayer, the angle of incidence for a given wavelength. As d increases, N_{eff} decreases. This is due to an increase in the absorption medium in the mirror.

Similarly N_{eff} is large for high photon energy and high angle of incidence. Reflector layer produces more absorption as the density of the medium is higher than the spacer. Hence it is a common practice it maintains the thickness of the reflector layer than that of the spacer layer in a bilayer. Figure 2.18 shows the effect of a number of bilayers on the peak reflectivity at the first Bragg peak of modeled W/B_4C multilayer mirror with d= 3.4 nm which is. Y-axis corresponds to the peak reflectivity at the first Bragg peak (90° in this case) of 0.183 keV X-rays. In this case, it is observed that the reflectivity initially increases as a number of bilayers increases and saturates close to 33 % at around 200 number of bilayers.

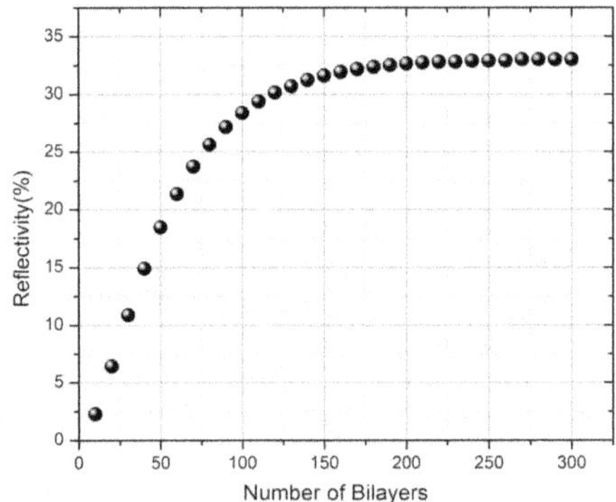

Figure 2.18: Effect of number of bi-layers on peak reflectivity at Bragg peak at 183 eV x-rays. This graph is calculated from modeling a W-B_4C multilayer mirror with $d = 34$ nm. The first Bragg peak occurs at 90°.

2.6.3   Effect of γ on X-ray reflectivity

γ gives the ratio of the thickness of the reflector layer (d_r) to the d. As reflectors have a high absorption coefficient due to their high density, in a bilayer, the layer thickness of the spacer is maintained larger than the thickness of the reflector layer. As a result, the maximum value of γ is restricted to 0.5 for all cases. The minimum value of γ is only limited by the minimum thickness of the reflector layer which can sufficiently reflect X-rays. Extremely small gamma values for thin multilayer mirrors are limited by the physical possibility to fabricate continuous sub-nanometer thick metallic layers. If the thickness of the metallic layer is smaller than the skin depth at a particular wavelength, the reflectivity is lowered. Figure 2.19 shows the simulated data of the change in Bragg peak reflectivity as a function γ. Y-axis of the first order Bragg peak reflectivity of a modeled $Ru - B_4C$ multilayer with d= 2.5 nm and N= 150. It is observed that the peak reflectivity is very low for small γ as the thickness of the reflector layer is too small to effectively reflect X-rays. At higher γ (> 0.4), the mirror becomes more absorbing as d_r increases. Peak values of γ also depend on the thickness of the multilayer mirror, and the angle of incidence.

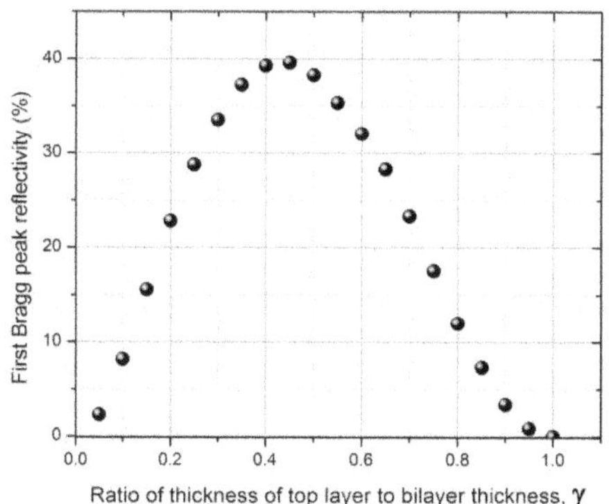

Figure 2.19: Effect of γ on reflectivity at first Bragg peak to a modelled Ru-B_4C multilayer mirror whose $d = 2.5$ nm with 150 repetitions.

From equation (2.40), when $\gamma= 0.5$, i.e. when the thickness of spacer and reflector are same, at Bragg condition ($\cos Qd =1$ and $Q=2\pi n /d$), the structure function reduces to (2.46),

$$|F(\theta_n)| = \left(\frac{d}{n\pi}\right)(\phi_r - \phi_s)sin(n\pi/2) \tag{2.46}$$

Equation (2.46) equals to zero when n is even. Substituting F=0 in equations (2.42), (2.43) and (2.41), the reflected intensity $I(\theta)$ =0. Hence when γ= 0.5, all even order Bragg peaks get suppressed. For a generic condition, from equation (2.40), the structure function at Bragg peaks $F(\theta_m)$ =0 when the term $cos(Q\gamma d)$ =0. Solving for this condition we get (2.47),

$$n\gamma = 1 \tag{2.47}$$

From the condition (2.47), it is noted that n^{th} of Bragg peak is suppressed when the value of γ is such that $n\gamma$ =1. Under this condition, the thickness of spacer and reflector layers are such that the partially reflected ray from reflector will be canceled out by the partially reflected ray from spacer component due to destructive interference. Figure 2.20 shows the simulated data of a modeled $Ru-B_4C$ multilayer mirror with d= 5 nm and N= 150. The response is calculated for an incident photon energy of 10 keV as a function of incident angle for different γ values. The suppression of higher order Bragg peaks can be observed for respective γ values which satisfy (2.47).

2.6.4 Choice of materials

Multilayer materials play an important role in maximizing the Bragg reflection. High the density and δ of the reflector material helps in high partial reflection from the layer whereas high β contributes to high absorption. Choice of materials also depends on the spectral range of operation. In the X-ray region, most of the materials have very strong absorption edges which behave as a strong absorbing

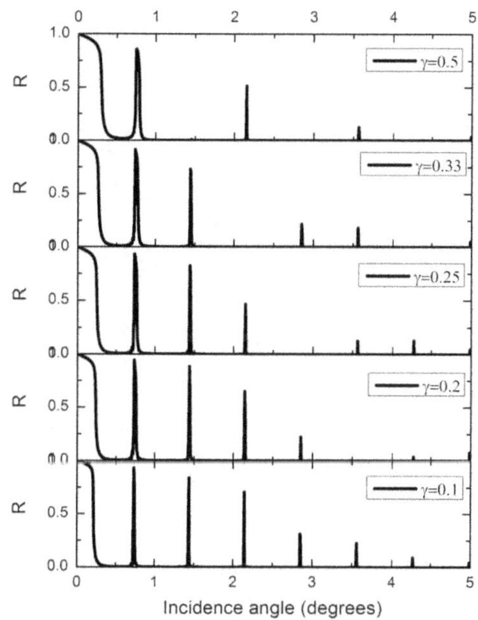

Figure 2.20: X-ray reflectivity curves showing the suppression of higher order Bragg peaks for different γ

medium instead of reflecting. At these regions the value of β is maximum hence, the overall reflectivity from the mirror is very low. Figure 2.21 shows the calculated Bragg reflectivity of multilayer mirrors with different reflector materials as a function a simple figure of merit which is given by $\rho\delta/(\beta \times atomicweight)$. This ratio gives the condition for a better choice of reflector material at a given wavelength. Spacers for all the cases is B_4C and the calculation is made at 0.18 keV with a period of a mirror at 3.4 nm. Y-axis is the first Bragg peak reflectivity which is at 90° in this case. Figure 2.21 indicates that, reflectivity is high for reflectors materials for high density and δ and low atomic weight and β.

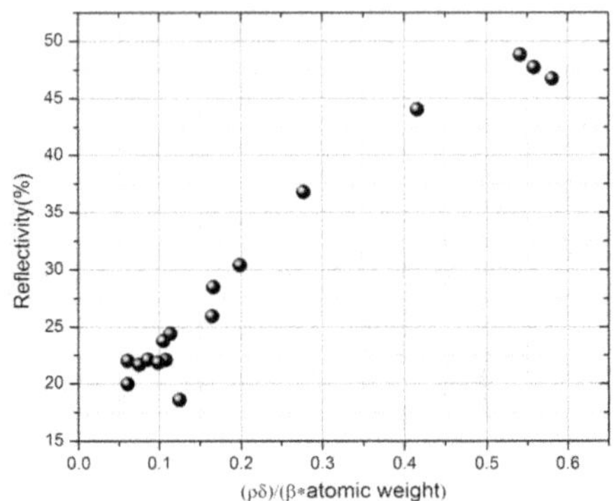

Figure 2.21: Bragg peak reflectivity of different materials as a function of $\left(\frac{\delta\rho}{\beta \times atomicweight}\right)$ of reflector layer. Spacer is B_4C for all cases. Reflectivities of these modelled mirror are calculated at first Bragg peak (at 90°) at 0.18 keV.

2.6.5 Resolving power of multilayer mirrors

Resolving power of multilayer mirrors is governed by the width of the Bragg peak. For a constant period multilayer mirror (d of all bilayers is maintained same), Bragg peaks are very narrow. The full width at half maximum (FWHM), $\Delta\theta_n$ of a Bragg peak is a function of a number of bilayers and the order of Bragg peak. For thick multilayer mirror, $\Delta\theta_n$ and the resolving power of Bragg peak R_n is given by (2.48) and (2.49) respectively [Michette, 1986]:

$$\Delta\theta_{n-thick} = (4/\sqrt{3}\pi)(A \tan\theta_n)/nN \tag{2.48}$$

$$R_{n-thick} = (\sqrt{3}\pi/4)nN/A \tag{2.49}$$

In case of thin multilayer mirrors (A < 0.4), $\Delta\theta_n$ and R_n are given by, (2.50) and (2.51) [Michette, 1986]

$$\Delta\theta_{n-thin} = 2[(ln2)/\pi]^{1/2}(\tan\theta_m)/nN \tag{2.50}$$

$$R_{n-thin} = 0.5(\pi/ln2)^{1/2}nN \simeq nN \tag{2.51}$$

Figure 2.22 shows the simulated reflectivity of the profile of W/B_4C multilayer mirrors with d= 3.5 nm at 2 keV as a function of incident angle. Bragg peak is much sharper for the sample with large layer pairs. These simulations are performed on modeled samples of uniform and sharp layer interfaces. However, in a physical system, layers are not sharp and have some interlayer diffusion which broadens the Bragg peak. The width of the Bragg peak is also very sensitive to the experimental conditions such as the divergence of the incident beam and the opening angle of the detector.

2.6.6 Surface roughness

As discussed in section 2.2.3, surface roughness severely affects the reflectivity of the X-ray mirror. However, for multilayer mirror where the reflectivity is contributed by all bilayers, the reflection at Bragg peaks is function interlayer roughness. From equation (2.19) and (2.20), the effect of roughness on reflectivity also depends on the incident angle and the wavelength of X-rays. Figure 2.23 shows the effect of roughness on the Bragg peak reflectivity at different energies and angles corresponding Bragg peaks (as indicated in the inset). These results are obtained for a modelled W/B_4C multilayer with d=2 nm and N=150. Reflectivity drops exponentially as the surface roughness increases. It is also observed the effect of roughness is larger at higher photon energies.

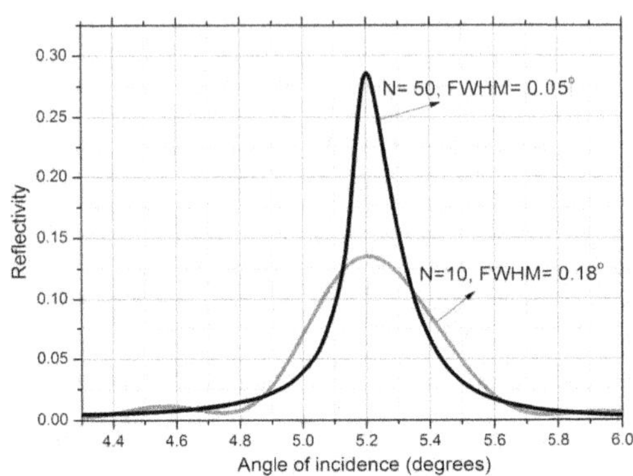

Figure 2.22: Reflectivity profile at 2 keV for two W/B_4C multilayer mirror mirrors with d= 3.5 nm and N= 10 and 50 respectively.

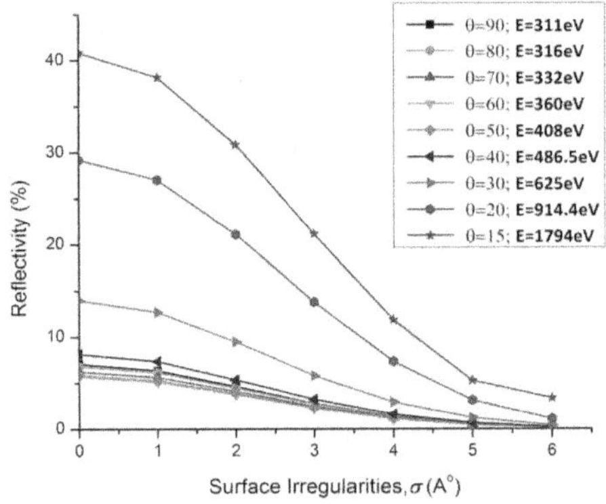

Figure 2.23: Influence of interlayer surface roughness of the mirror on the reflectivity of W/B_4C multilayer mirror with d= 2 nm and N=150.

2.7 Summary

In this chapter, we have presented the theory and simulated results on the X-ray reflection from thin films. We have presented a comprehensive discussion on the effects of various parameters like the coating thickness, roughness, X-ray wavelength, angle of incidence on the reflection efficiency. We have also discussed in detail regarding various optical design for X-ray imaging telescope and concentrator optics. Design and working principle of multilayer mirrors is discussed. Simulated results of the effects of several design parameters are presented in this chapter.

Chapter 3

Fabrication and testing of multilayer mirrors

The process of depositing thin films of materials are broadly classified into two parts: Physical Vapour Deposition (PVD) and Chemical Vapour Deposition (CVD). In PVD techniques, the material goes from the condensed phase to the vapor phase to gets deposited as a thin film on the substrate back to condensed phase. Deposition techniques like evaporation and sputtering are classified as PVD techniques. In CVD, the substrate is exposed to one or more volatile materials which react and decompose on to the substrate. CVD is preferably performed in a vacuum and the volatile by-products formed by the chemical reactions are later removed by the gas flow.

3.1   Thin film deposition techniques

3.1.1   Thermal evaporation

Thermal evaporation is the oldest PVD technique which is used to deposit thin films on a substrate. In this technique, the material to be deposited is kept in ultra-high vacuum (10^{-6} Torr) and heated to temperatures to vaporize the material. A substrate is placed in these vapors which then condenses a thin layer of material. In this technique,target materials are heated to high temperatures (a few thousands for metals). This technique is not useful for depositing alloy materials as different compounds need different temperatures to vaporize. Thin films fabricated using this technique usually undergo large thermal stresses.

3.1.2   Electron beam (e- beam) evaporation

Electron beam or e-beam evaporation is PVD technique which allows fast deposition of thin films. This is similar to thermal evaporation but uses a high-current electron gun to produces vapors of the coating material. Highly focused e- beam produces a very localized rise in temperatures which leads to local evaporation of the target material. Deposition rate can be measured in-situ by placing a piezoelectric quartz crystal which changes its natural frequency of oscillation as a function of the amount of deposited material.

3.1.3   Sputtering

In the sputtering technique, particles are ejected from the material as a result of the bombardment of energetic particles (gas ions). These particles are then deposited on to a substrate and form a thin film. The properties of the emitted particles depend on the kinetic energy of the bombarding ions, their angle of incidence and the target material geometry. Sputtering can be done by ion beams (Ion beam sputtering), high power pulsed Lasers (Pulsed Laser deposition) and high power direct current (DC) and radio frequency alternating cycle current (RF-AC) sources.

DC Sputtering: Figure 3.1 shows the schematic of a DC sputtering system for metallic layer deposition. A substrate connected to a positive potential (anode) is placed in front of a target material which is connected to a negative potential (cathode). Coating chamber is maintained at low pressure ($\sim 10^-3$ Torr) of pure Ar or Kr gas which is used as the sputtered gas. When high electric field ($\sim 10,000V$) applied to the system, plasma is generated in the chamber. Plasma consists of electrons and positive ions of sputtered gas. Sputtered gas is usually an inert gas as other gases like Oxygen and Nitrogen will chemically react with the target material. Helium and Neon are not usually preferred as they require relatively large power to create plasma . Ar is the most commonly used sputtered gas. Positive ions of sputtered gas hit the negatively charged target material with great force and remove some material. The number of target atoms released by each sputtered ion is called the sputtering yield which is a function of target materials, applied power, the pressure inside the coating chamber and the angle of impact of the sputtered ion to the target material. Atoms from the target come towards the substrate with some kinetic energy and gets deposited as a thin film. These atoms can also cause re-sputtering from the deposited substrate if the kinetic energy of the atom is strong enough to break the bonding of the layer [Greene, 2017]. Figure 3.2 shows the schematic of cases of sputtering and re-sputtering.

RF Sputtering DC sputtering technique produces smooth, thin and uniform metallic layers. However, this technique is not useful for the deposition of the insulator layer. When the target material is an insulator, Ar ions initially sputter

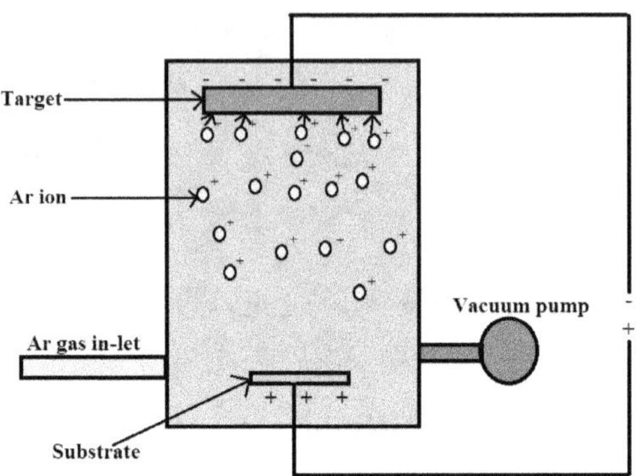

Figure 3.1: Schematic of DC magnetron sputtering mechanism to deposit thin films

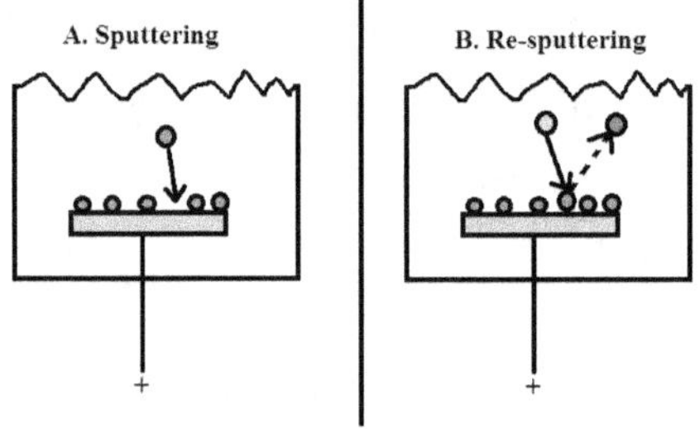

Figure 3.2: Schematic of process representing Left (A): Sputtering process for thin film deposition. Right (B): Re-sputtering where deposited layers get sputtered back to vapour.

the material for a short period. Over time, the surface of the target will be positively charged. Whereas in the case of metals, the negative power supply will discharge the positive surface of the target. But in the case of an insulator, the surface remains positive which stops further sputtering of positively charged Ar ions. Figure 3.3 shows the schematic of DC sputtering of insulator where the surface becomes positive repelling the positively charged Ar ions.

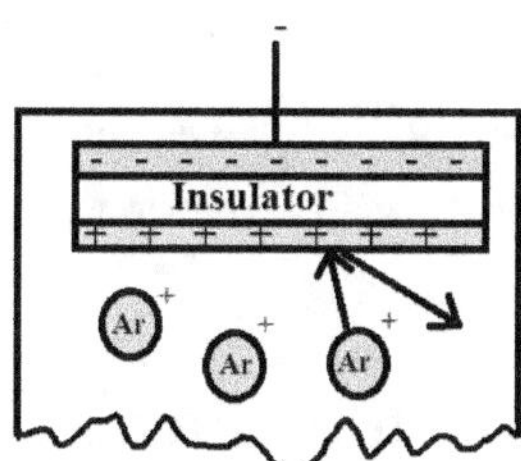

Figure 3.3: Schematic of DC sputtering system for insulator target. The outer surface of the target becomes positive resisting positively charges Ar ions from sputtering.

This problem is addressed by using Radio Frequency (RF) AC power supply. In RF sputtering systems, the power supply is in AC mode with typically 75% positive and 25% negative cycle. Alternating positive and negative power supplies to target help in discharging the insulator target allowing Ar ion to continuously hit the target material for sputtering.

Uniformity of layers: Uniformity of the layer deposition on the substrate depends on the relative sizes of substrate and target and the distance between the target and substrate. Uniformity of layers can be improved by increasing the distance between the target and the substrate. However, this makes the system huge. Rotating the wafer during deposition can improve uniformity. But is not feasible in all coating chambers. Collimators can be used in front of the target material which allows only the particles traveling in a straight path to get deposited on the substrate. This technique significantly decreases the deposition rate. One of the most commonly used technique to increase the uniformity and deposition efficiency of sputtering is by using a magnetic field to direct the plasma. Such systems are called "magnetron sputtering" system [Hull, 1921]. In magnetron sputtering

system, the magnetic field is configured parallel to the target surface. This will
not only increases the uniformity of deposition but also increase the probability of
atom-electron collision and constrains the motion of secondary electrons.

3.2 Fabrication of multilayer mirrors by magnetron sputtering

Magnetron sputtering technique is one of the most popular techniques to fabricate multilayer mirrors as they produce sharp interfaces and thin layers. We have
fabricated W/B_4C multilayer mirrors using magnetron sputtering system at Raja
Ramanna Center for Advanced Technology (RRCAT) [Nayak et al., 2012], Indore,
India. Since multilayer mirrors typically have both metallic and non-metallic (insulator) layers, the sputtering system has both DC as well RF power supply. Figure
3.4 shows the schematic of the magnetron sputtering system used to fabricate
multilayer mirrors.

The system consists of two targets, one for spacer material (RF power supply)
and other is for reflector material (DC power supply). A substrate is placed on a
translating stage to form spacer and reflector targets. The system is evacuated to
ultra-high vacuums of about 3×10^{-8} m Bar. A pure Argon (Ar) gas is sent to the
chamber as a sputtering gas until the pressure reaches 5×10^{-3} m Bar. When a
high voltage of DC and RF is applied to reflector and spacer targets respectively,
plasma is formed inside the coating chamber. The power supply is varied according
to the type of material and the desired deposition rate. In the system we used
to fabricate W/B_4C multilayers, we haveused 70 W DC to Tungsten and 700 W
RF to B_4C target. When stable plasma is formed inside the coating chamber,
the positively charged Ar ions bombard with the target material and produces

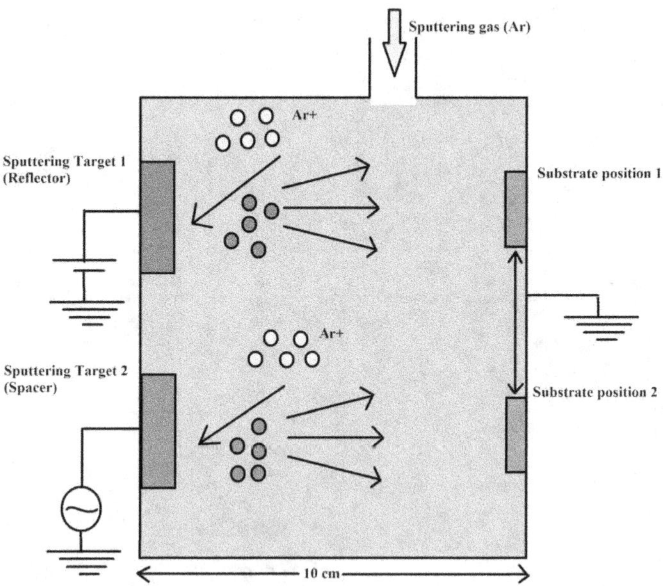

Figure 3.4: Schematic of magnetron sputtering system for multilayer deposition.

the vapors of respective materials. The substrate is placed in front of the target material for a pre-calibrated time whose layer has to be deposited with a certain thickness. Substrate alternatively moves from spacer and reflector target for the deposition of alternating layers. Figure 3.5 shows the picture of the magnetron sputtering system at RRCAT which is used to fabricate all the multilayer mirrors discussed in this thesis.

3.3 Testing of multilayer mirrors

Characterization of multilayer mirrors is done by measuring the X-ray reflectivity, surface roughness, period of bilayers number of layers pairs and the density of

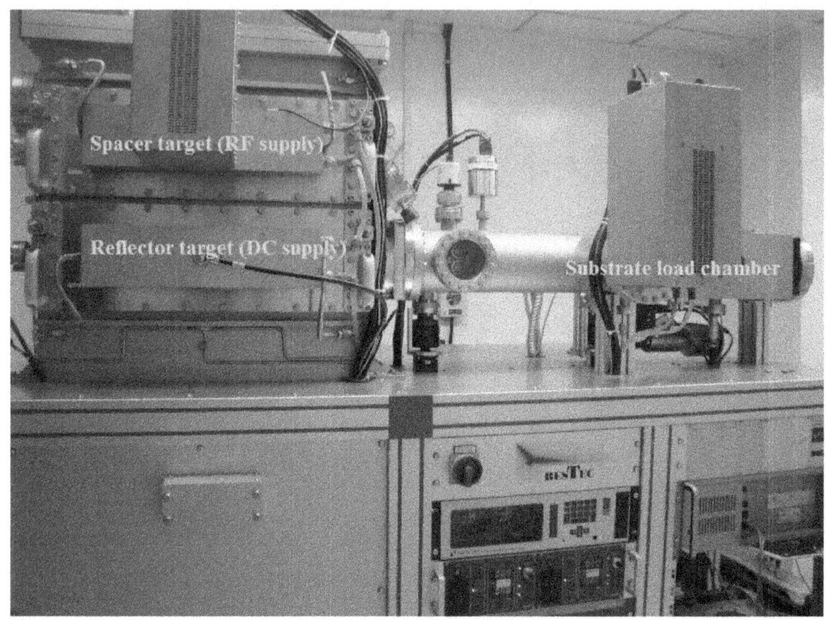

Figure 3.5: Picture of magnetron sputtering system at RRCAT which is used to fabricate all multilayer mirrors discussed in this thesis.

the material of the thin film. Standard optical profilometers very precisely give the surface roughness of the top layer of the film. But for multilayer mirrors, the interlayer roughness plays a major role in governing the overall reflectivity of the mirror. Transmission electron microscopes (TEM) can be used to characterize both thickness of each layer as well as the interlayer roughness. However, the resolution of TEM is poor to image ultra-short period multilayer mirrors. TEM technique also destroys the sample which makes it not feasible to test on the mirrors which have to used for further applications. Atomic force microscope (AFM) is widely used for precise measurement of the roughness of the sample. However, AFM also gives the roughness measure of the top layer. While many other material and optical characterization techniques are available for measuring the surface and material properties of mirrors, none of them are optimized to study all the parameters of multilayer mirrors. X-ray reflectivity (XRR) measurement technique is the most widely used technique for not only measuring the absolute reflection efficiency of mirrors but also gives the estimate of all design parameters like the period of bilayers, number of bilayers, interlayer roughness, density of materials, etc.

3.3.1   X-ray reflectivity (XRR) technique

X-ray reflectivity (XRR) technique is a non-destructive technique of measuring the design parameters as well as the absolute reflectivity of multilayer mirrors. Since this technique is non-destructive, measurements can be made even on mirrors with further applications. A basic XRR setup consists of an X-ray gun, sample holder and an X-ray detector. Narrow slits are used both at source and detector ends to restrict the X-ray beam. For X-ray reflectivity measurements, a perfectly aligned system is scanned across angles (θ) from the required range such that the source and the detector maintain $\theta - 2\theta$ at all times. Schematic of a basic XRR setup is shown in the figure 3.6. To maintain $\theta - 2\theta$ conditions either the source and detector are moved using a goniometer keeping sample stationary or by tilting the sample and moving the detector by keeping the source stationery.

XRR setup using a synchrotron radiation source facility in beamlines adopt the stationary source and movable sample detector configuration. Laboratory XRR setups which use monochromatic X-ray sources have a goniometer arrangement of source and detector with a stationary sample. Figure 3.7 shows the picture of a laboratory XRR setup at RRCAT which uses Copper (Cu) target to produces 8.047 keV (Cu-kα) line emission.

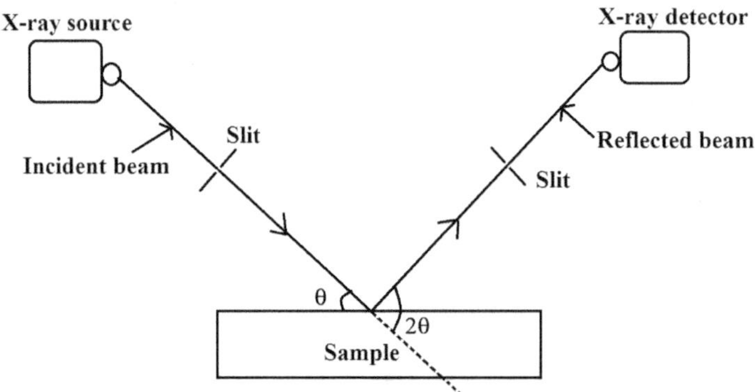

Figure 3.6: Schematic of basic XRR setup

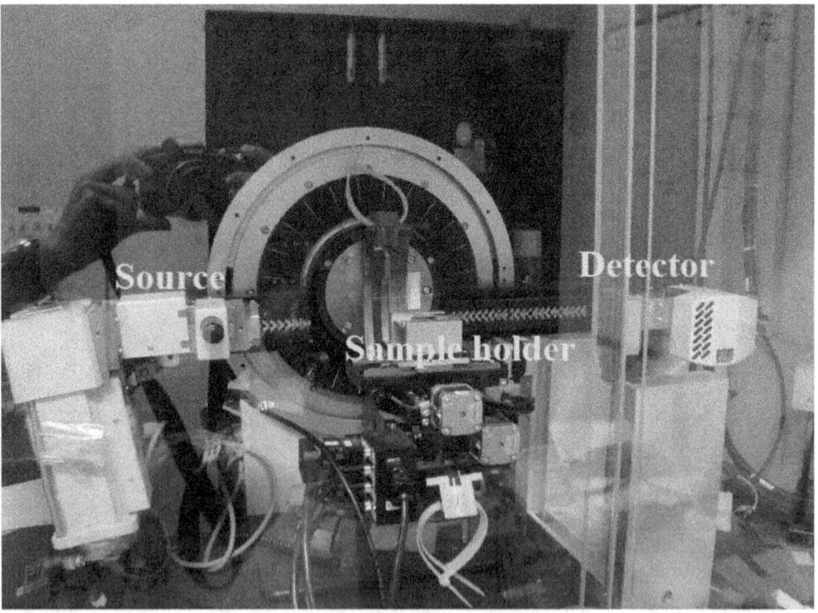

Figure 3.7: Picture of a laboratory XRR setup at RRCAT which uses Copper target to produce 8.047 keV (Cu-kα) line emission.

3.3.2 Determination of multilayer parameters using XRR data

A typical XRR data consist of reflectivity as a function of the angle of incidence at a monochromatic X-ray source. Figure 3.8 shows the typical XRR data of modeled multilayer mirrors similar design parameters with different roughness. This data can be fitted to multilayer mirror models to extract parameters.

Determination of 'N' by Kiessig fringes

Kiessig fringes are formed between two Bragg peaks as a result of secondary reflections between the layers. A number of Kiessig fringes between grazing incidence peak and the first Bragg peak is given by $N - 2$. Hence by measuring a number of Kiessig fringes, the number of bilayers in a multilayer mirror can be determined. However, this technique cannot be efficiently used for a large number of bilayers as the angular resolution of the measurement is smaller than the width of Keissig peak.

Determination of 'd' by the position of Bragg peaks

From the Bragg's law, the relation between the position of the mth order Bragg peak, the wavelength of incident light and the period of the bi-layer is established. Hence by calculating the angle at which the peak reflectivity of a Bragg peak occurs, the period of multilayer mirrors can be determined for a monochromatic source

Determination of surface roughness 'σ' by peak reflectivity

While the number of kiessig fringes is an indicator of a number of bi-layers, the slope at which the intensity of these oscillations decay gives the surface roughness

of a multilayer mirror. This, in turn, affects the peak reflectivity of the Bragg
peak. Surface roughness can be quantitatively determined by fitting the measured
data from XRR test in software like IMD or Parratt which are virtual laboratories
for modeling MCMs and conducting XRR tests.

Determination of density 'ρ' from critical angle

Density of material in a thin film deposited by sputtering is different from the
density of the target material. True density of the coated material can be found
by measuring the critical angle from XRR test results. The critical angle of total
reflection gives the density of the top layer. The density of interlayer mediate
layers can be determined by fitting the peak reflectivity and the contrast of Kiessig
oscillations.

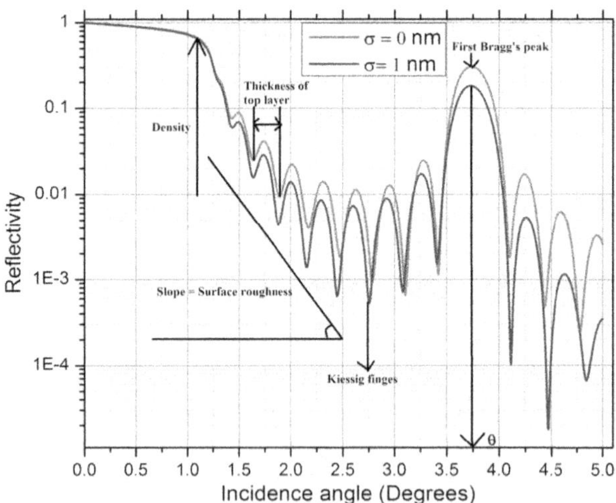

Figure 3.8: Calculated reflectivity profiles of two modelled multilayers using IMD
software. This data is useful for determining several design parameters of multilayer mirrors.

3.4 Calibration of magnetron sputtering system

Parameters like the power supply, Ar pressure, the distance between the target and the substrate, exposure time of substrate to sputtering plasma etc., affects the uniformity, thickness, and roughness of the deposited layer. All parameters are optimized in the system to produce smooth and uniform multilayers. The exposure time of substrate to target material plasma is varied according to thickness requirements. Uniformity of coating depends on the size of the target. In the system we have used to fabricate the samples, the target is 30 cm × 5 cm. Hence the sputtering is more uniform in shorter dimension. To test the uniformity we have fabricated a test W/B_4C sample with 20 bilayers. Ar pressure, power and exposure time of the system is optimized to fabricate sample of thickness 1.6 nm. Sample (3 cm × 3 cm) is placed at the center of the substrate holder. After fabrication, the sample is tested for X-ray reflectivity at 6 different positions both across horizontal as well as the vertical axis. Figure 3.9 shows the schematic of the sample on a sample holder placed in the coating chamber. Lines numbering 1 to 6 are the approximate positions where XRR measurement is conducted. Figure 3.10 shows the XRR results at all positions as marked in figure 3.9. From the figure 3.10 it is observed that the period of the multilayer mirror has changed across the sample. It is noted that the period of multilayers is mostly unchanged along horizontal axis. Whereas the period changed in the order of 0.2 nm from top to bottom of the mirror. This shows the coating is more uniformity can be correlated to the dimensions of the sputtering target. Table 3.1 shows the measured periods of the multilayer mirror at various positions. It is also observed that the Bragg peak reflectivity and the intensity of the Kiessig oscillations are also changed at different positions.

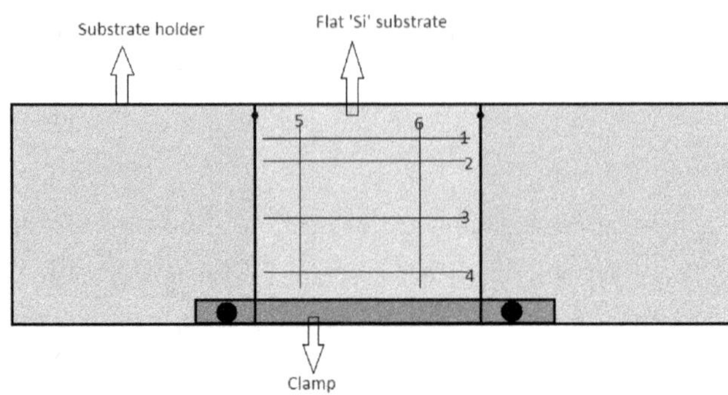

Figure 3.9: Schematic of the substrate holder with thin substrate mounted on it which is placed inside the coating chamber. Approximated locations are numbered where the XRR data are collected.

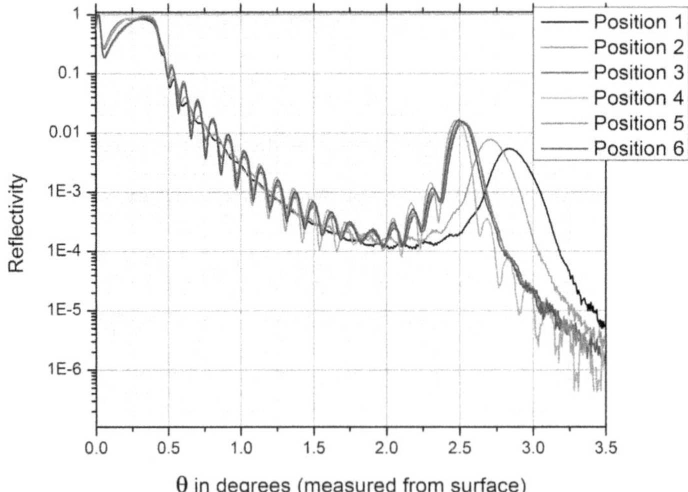

Figure 3.10: XRR results conducted using 8.047 keV lab source at all 6 positions on the coated mirror. Deviation in Bragg peak is observed for positions 1 and 2 which indicates a change in the period of multilayer mirrors.

We have also observed that the deposition rate is fast when the distance between the substrate and target is small. The power supply can also be varied to

Table 3.1: calculated bilayer period of multilayer mirror at various position.

Position	d (nm)
1	1.59
2	1.64
3	1.77
4	1.80
5	1.77
6	1.76

change the deposition rate. However, the relation between the power-used and the deposition rate is not linear over a wide range of values.

3.5 Sample preparation of W/B_4C multilayer mirrors using magnetron sputtering system

W/B_4C multilayer mirrors of different periods and a different number of layer pairs are fabricated. Table 3.2 gives the specifications of magnetron sputtering system for fabrication these mirrors. These specifications are kept unchanged except for the "number of cycles" for fabricating mirrors with different specifications. A number of cycles are varied according to the thickness requirement of each layer. As the number of cycles increased, the thickness of the layer is increased. A DC power supply is applied to the Tungsten target and a RF- AC with a positive DC bias is applied to the B_4C. Positive DC bias increases the percentage of positive voltage power supply to increase the efficiency of the sputtering process. To increase the uniformity of the coating, a narrow slit is placed in-front of the substrate which allows only collimated particles of material to get deposited on the substrate. The substrate is scanned across the slit for uniform coverage. Scanning speed is different for Tungsten and B_4C targets as the rate of deposition are different. The

number of cycles indicates the number of times the substrate is scanned across the
slit for one layer deposition. This parameter is varied as per the period of bilayers.
The vacuum in the coating chamber is maintained at the level of 1×10^{-7} mbar
before injecting pure Ar gas. Ar gas is injected till the pressure increases up to
approximately 3×10^{-3} mbar. The pressure usually increases during the sputtering
process to approximately to 1×10^{-2} mbar due to the formation of plasma.

Table 3.2: Magnetron sputtering system specifications for fabricating W/B_4C multilayer mirrors

Parameter	W (Tungsten)	B_4C
Power (Watts)	70 (DC)	700 (RF)
DC-Bias (V)	-	1000
Scanning speed (mm/s)	9.2	1.2
No. of cycles (d-3.5 nm)	2	7
No. of cycles (d-5.5 nm)	3	13

A number of W/B_4C multilayer mirrors are fabricated with a period ranging
from 1.5 nm to 5.8 nm and a number of bilayers varying from 50 to 300. Table
3.3 gives the list of all the fabricated W/B_4C multilayer mirrors with their specifications and the reflectivity at 8 keV which is measured immediately after the
fabrication.

3.6 Multi-wavelength reflectivity analysis of multilayer mirrors

The reflectivity of multilayer mirrors depends on the optical constants of the materials of bilayers. We have conducted the multi-wavelength reflectivity analysis of a
W/B_4C sample with period 1.9 nm and 170 number of bilayers. Figure 3.11 [Panini

Table 3.3: Specifications of all mirrors for testing and the reflectivity at 8 at keV
which is measured immediately after coating

Sl. No	d(nm)	N	R@ 8ekV
1	1.5	300	10.2
2	1.6	300	13.8
3	1.9	170	19.1
4	3.3	70	30.6
5	3.3	70	30.2
6	3.3	70	24.2
7	3.35	70	26.1
8	3.55	700	18.7
9	4.4	50	38.7
10	5.22	50	20.3
11	5.4	50	24.7
12	5.8	50	25.4

et al., 2018] gives the measured reflectivity data from 9 keV to 16 keV. These measurements are made using the beamline (BL-16) [Tiwari et al., 2012] of the Indus -2 synchrotron radiation facility, RRCAT, Indore. It is observed that as the energy of the incident photon increases, the Bragg peak angle decreases. It is also observed that the critical angle of reflection reduces as the energy increases.

The maximum Bragg reflectivity varies with the energy of the incident photon. Figure 3.12 (data in red) shows the measured maximum reflectivity at the first Bragg peak of the sample as a function of incident photon energy. It is observed that the reflectivity of the mirror drops rapidly between the range from 10 keV to 12 keV. This is due to the presence of an absorption edge of Tungsten in that region. At the absorption edge, the layer material becomes more absorbing than reflecting which lowers the reflectivity. The imaginary term in the complex reflective index gives the absorption coefficient. In figure 3.12 the data in blue represents the reciprocal of the absorption coefficient of Tungsten (imaginary part of the refractive index). A clear correlation can be observed between the reflectivity and the inverse of the absorption coefficient of Tungsten.

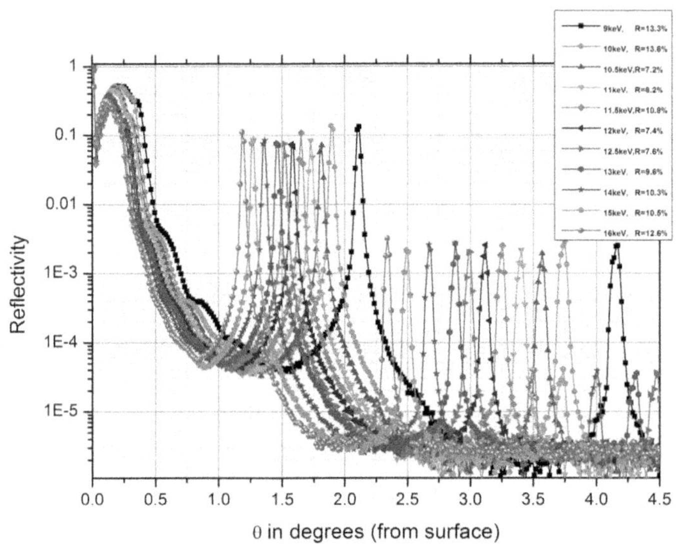

Figure 3.11: Measured hard X-ray reflectivity data of multilayer mirror of sample with period 1.9 nm and 170 number of bilayers from 9 keV to 16 keV. As the energy of incident photon increases, the angle of the Bragg peak decreases.

Resolution of multilayer mirrors: From equation (2.51) of chapter 2, it is observed that the resolution of multilayer mirror is a function of photon energy. As the energy of the incident photon increases, the FWHM of the Bragg peak becomes smaller and thus improving the resolution of a multilayer mirror. Figure 3.13 shows the measured FWHM at first Bragg peak of the mirror measured at various energies.

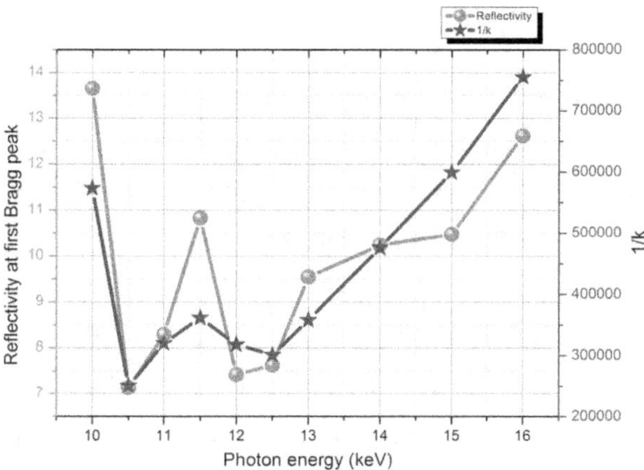

Figure 3.12: Measured reflectivity at first Bragg peak of a sample with period 1.9 nm and 170 layer pairs as a function of photon energy (red). The reflectivity data are over plotted alongside the inverse of absorption coefficient of Tungsten. Reflectivity varies inversely with the absorption coefficient of the reflector material.

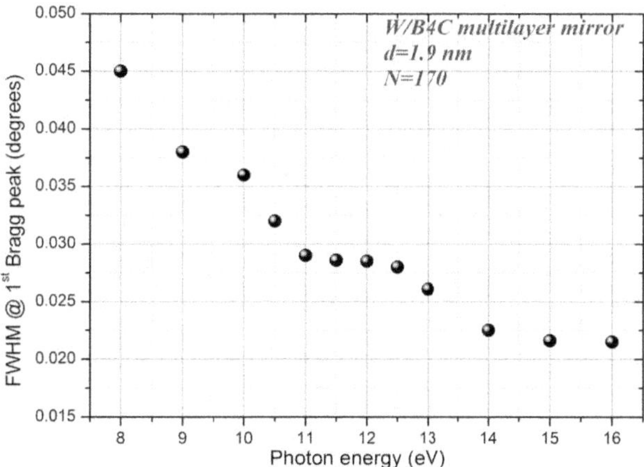

Figure 3.13: Measured FWHM of W/B_4C sample with period 1.9 nm and 170 layers pairs as a function of the photon energy.

3.7 Summary

W/B_4C multilayer mirrors are fabricated using magnetron sputtering technique. We have characterised and optimized the sputtering system to fabricate multilayer mirrors with very smooth interface. Several multilayer mirrors with varied period from 15 nm - 58 nm and number of bilayers from 50 to 300 are fabricated and tested. We have conducted multi-wavelength reflectivity measurements from 8 keV to 16 keV using synchrotron beamline. We have observed that the resolving power of the mirror increases with the photon energy. We have also observed that the short period multilayer mirrors have higher resolution while the large period multilayers have higher reflection efficiency.

Chapter 4

Thermal and temporal stability of W/B_4C multilayer mirrors

Multilayer mirrors developed for space applications has to withstand the dynamic environmental conditions experienced by a satellite. Due to the absence of an atmosphere, the temperature difference between the sunlit (day) and earth occulted (night) regions in the low earth orbit, is large. A satellite in a low earth orbit experiences rapid temperature variations ranging from $\sim +50^o$ C (sunlit) to $\sim -40^o$ C (earth shadow) over a 90-minute orbit. Hence multilayer mirrors used for these applications should with-stand such rapid temperature variations. W/B_4C multilayers mirrors are know to form a smooth ans stable interface structures [Jankowski and Makowiecki, 1991], [Jankowski et al., 1989], [Gutman, 1994]. Weak chemical interactions between Tungsten (W) and Boron Carbide (B_4C) helps to lower the interlayer diffusion between the layers [Jankowski and Makowiecki, 1991], [Gutman, 1994], [Okada et al., 1994], [Jankowski. et al., 1990]. While W/B_4C multilayer mirrors are known to be stable for high temperature ($\sim +800^o$ C) [Rao et al., 2013] applications, rapid temperature gradients could affect structural integrity due to differential expansion/contraction between bi-layers. We studied the long-time stability and the effects of rapid temperature variations on the structural and optical properties of W/B_4C multilayer mirrors with different periods. The multilayers with periods ranging from 5.4 nm to 1.6 nm are used for this study. Large period multilayer is used for high reflectivity applications whereas short period multilayer mirrors provide high spectral resolution and can operate at relatively larger angles. We have thermal cycled several sets of multilayer mirrors with different periods over 1 day, 3 days, and 10 days. Variations in structure and reflectivity of these mirrors arising from cycling are monitored with hard X-ray reflectivity (HXR) measurements using a laboratory-based X-ray source with a copper target, scanning electron microscopy (SEM) and soft X-ray reflectivity (SXR) using the BL-3 beamline [Modi et al., 2019] at Indus-2 synchrotron radiation facility.

4.1   Long time stability of multilayer mirrors

For a typical decade-long gestation period to develop space payloads and a minimum of 5 years in orbit, it is crucial to limit performance degradation of multilayers over time. Over the course of the mission, variations in mirror characteristics have to be folded into periodic corrections to the pre-launch system response. Hence a clear understanding of the factors that contribute to loss of the performance of the optics while on ground and in space is essential to further optimize choice of materials, multilayer design and in creating in-orbit predictive models. We have addressed the ageing effect by studying the performance of three W/B_4C multilayers with period 1.9, 3.4 and 5.8 nm over two years since fabrication.

Reflectivity at the first Bragg peak of all the mirrors remained mostly unchanged with a little degradation during the first few months. Figure 4.1 shows the measured X-ray reflectivity data of sample with period 1.9 nm over two years. Figure 4.2 shows the peak reflectivity of the first Bragg peak of the mirror as a function of time. A small drop in reflectivity is observed over the initial few months and then the reflectivity is mostly unchanged over time. A slight change in the peak reflectivity can also occur due to changes in experimental setup. Figure 4.3 and 4.4 show the reflectivity data of samples with period 3.4 and 5.8 nm respectively at various times since manufacture. By fitting the model to the data, it is observed that the structural parameters like the interface width of layers, period and thickness ratio remained stable during this period. It is noteworthy to mention that for HXR measurements, different angular step size $\Delta\theta$ are used (see Table 4.1) for measurements at different times using different reflectometers. It is to be noted that the peak reflectivity at Bragg peaks is highly sensitive to $\Delta\theta$ of the measurement. For example, by changing angular step size from 0.015^o to 0.025^o, the first order Bragg peak of the sample with period 3.4 changes from 51% to 30% with same structural parameters. *So, the drop in reflectivity for the sample during the first 11 months is mainly due undersampling the measurement data.* The density of materials in thin films usually differs from that of their bulk density. Density variation from bulk is large for short period multilayers. For a sample with d=1.9 nm, the density of W layer is obtained as 16.2 g/cc (bulk density is 19.3) and the density of B_4C is 4.1 g/cc (bulk density is 2.52). For larger period multilayer mirrors, the densities of the materials are closer to the actual bulk values. The bulk density of material on the top surface affects the critical angle of reflection and the contrast in the densities of a bi-layer affects the peak reflectivity of the Bragg peak. The bulk densities for the materials in the mirrors are determined by fitting corresponding features from the measured data.

A systematic growth in the top contamination layer thickness and its interface width over time is observed from the reflectivity profile. The presence of the contamination layer can be inferred by observing the oscillations in the reflectivity data between the critical angle and the first Bragg peak. Contamination of the layer can be due to the oxidation of the top layer material in the mirror. From the data, it is observed that oscillations increase over time for the mirror with the period of 1.9 nm. This indicates the growth of an oxidation layer. As the thickness of the oxidation layer increases, the frequency of oscillation increases. It is also observed that as the period of multilayer increases the oxidation layer becomes less prominent. For large period multilayer mirror (d-5.8 nm, figure 4.4), no oscillations are observed even after two years from manufacture. Table 4.1 shows the measured 1st peak reflectivity at 8.047 keV of all three samples at different times. The table also provides the best-fit parameters to the measured HXR data of multilayers obtained using IMD software [Windt, 1998]. Here, t_c and σ_c are the thickness and interface width of the top contamination layer, respectively.

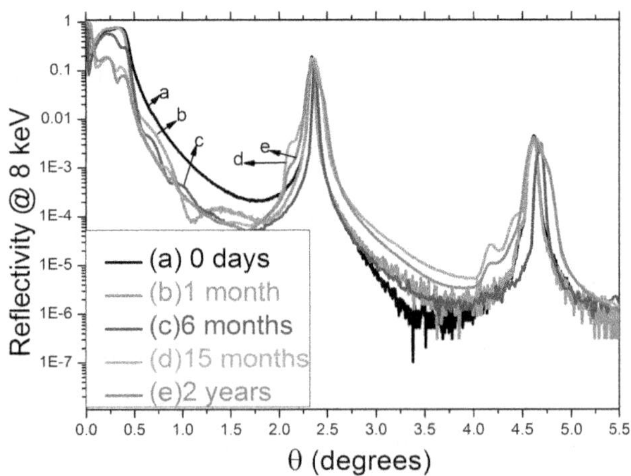

Figure 4.1: Measured reflectivity profile of the sample with period 1.9 nm at 8.047 keV at various times since manufacture. The variation near critical angle for 15 months and 2 years data is due to absence knife edge during measurement.

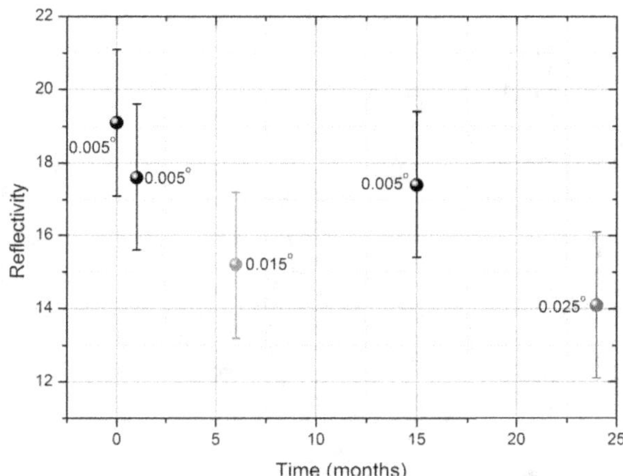

Figure 4.2: Variation of reflectivity at first Bragg peak of sample with period 1.9 nm at 8.047 keV over time. These measurements are conducted over time by using different experimental set-ups. The angular resolutions usded for each measurement is presented nest tot he data point. These respective angular resolutions are considered for fitting to determine the structural parameters of the mirror.

Figure 4.5 the thickness of the oxidation layer as a function of time for multilayer mirrors with different thickness. Formation of the contamination layer is due to the oxidation of Tungsten present in the mirror. Oxidation of B_4C is prominent only at very high temperatures ($> 500^oC$) and is mostly stable with oxygen at room temperatures. However, all samples are fabricated with B_4C being the outer-most surface which is known to have high chemical stability in standard atmospheric conditions. However, for short period multilayers, the top B_4C layer can be quasi-discontinuous which allows the bottom W layer to interact with the atmosphere

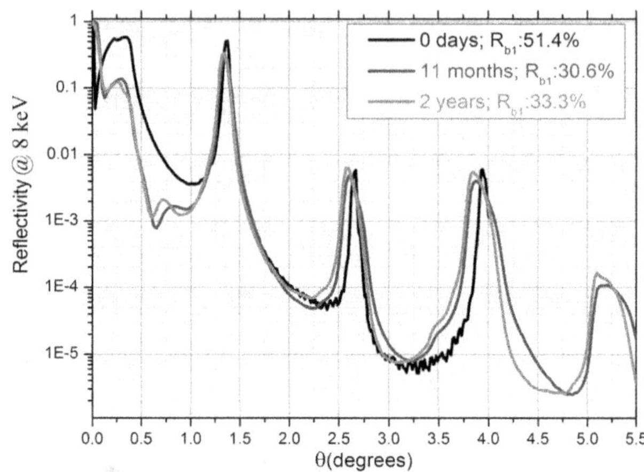

Figure 4.3: Measured reflectivity profile of the sample with period 3.4 nm at 8.047 keV at various times since manufacture.

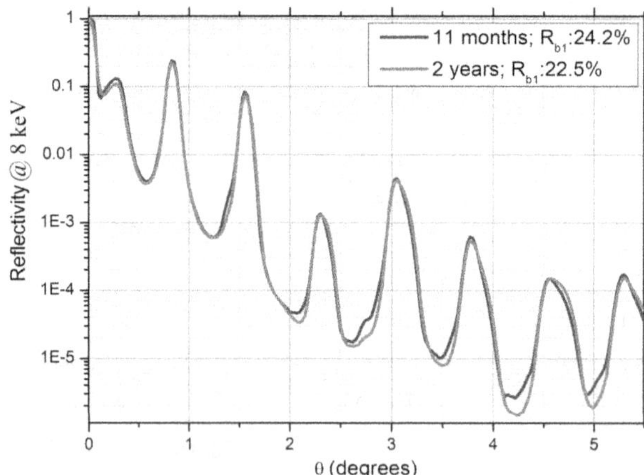

Figure 4.4: Measured reflectivity profile of the sample with period 5.8 nm at 8.047 keV at various times since manufacture.

and get oxidized. But as the period of multilayer increases, B_4C layer becomes more continuous and completely shields the W layer from direct contact with the

Table 4.1: Measured first order Bragg peak reflectivity and fitted parameters of three multilayer samples measured at 8.047 keV at various times. R_{1B}, σ_w and σ_{B_4C} are reflectivity of first order Bragg peak, interface width of W and interface width of B_4C respectively. t_c and σ_c are the thickness and the roughness of the contamination layer.

Parameter	R_{1B} (%)	$\Delta\theta$ (degrees)	σ_{B_4C} (nm)	σ_W (nm)	t_c (nm)	σ_c (nm)
d-1.9 nm, N- 170, Γ =0.45						
0 days	19.1±1	0.005	0.46 ±0.04	0.56 ±0.05	0	-
1 month	17.6 ±0.9	0.005	0.47 ±0.04	0.57 ±0.05	5.9 ±0.3	0.5 ±0.02
6 months	15.2 ±1	0.015	0.47 ±0.04	0.57 ±0.05	12.5 ±0.75	2.1 ±0.1
15 months	17.4 ±0.9	0.005	0.48 ±0.04	0.58 ±0.06	12.5 ±0.62	2.5 ±0.12
2 years	14.1 ±1.5	0.025	0.48 ±0.05	0.58 ±0.06	12.5 ±1.2	3.1 ±0.15
d-3.35 nm, N- 70, Γ =0.4						
0 days	51.4 ±2.5	0.015	0.32 ±0.03	0.62 ±0.06	0	-
11 months	30.6 ±2.1	0.025	0.43 ±0.04	0.72 ±0.07	2.8 ±0.2	2 ±0.1
2 years	33.6 ±2.3	0.025	0.42 ±0.04	0.71 ±0.07	3.2 ±0.3	2.5 ±0.32
d-5.8 nm, N- 50, Γ =0.4						
11 months	24.2 ±2.4	0.05	0.46 ±0.05	0.82 ±0.08	0	-
2 years	24.1 ±2.4	0.05	0.48 ±0.05	0.83 ±0.08	0	-

atmosphere. Hence the oxidation layer thickness reduces with the increase in the multilayer period; no oxidation layer was observed for large period multilayers. Figure 4.6 shows the toy model explaining the formation of an oxidation layer for short period multilayers. In the case of short-period multilayers, the micro roughness on the thin films causes makes the layer discontinuous exposing the bottom Tungsten layer to the atmosphere. For large period multilayer, large thickness layers can sufficiently mask the inner layers from the atmospheric oxygen. We have observed such discontinuous regions on soft period multilayer mirrors using Scanning Electron Microscope (SEM) and obtained the spectra of at those regions. Figure 4.7 shows the SEM data of a discontinuous top surface region of the sample with period 1.9 nm and the corresponding spectra taken by energy dispersion spectroscopy (EDX) is given below. From the spectra, the presence of Tungsten and Oxygen are evident at the selected region.

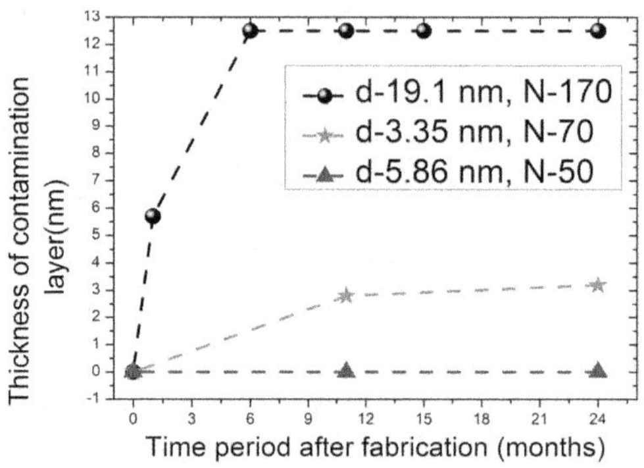

Figure 4.5: The growth of oxidation layer over time for samples with three different periods.

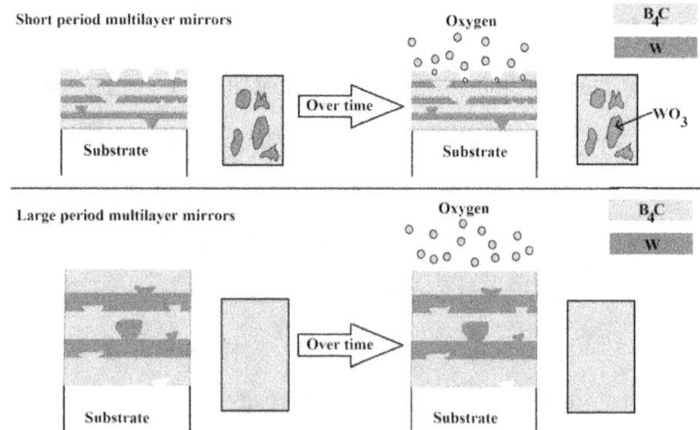

Figure 4.6: A toy model representing explaining the formation of contamination layer for short period multilayer mirrors.

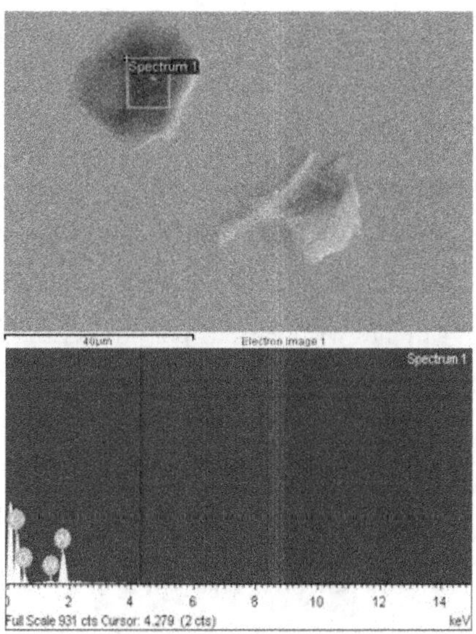

Figure 4.7: SEM data of sample with period 1.9 nm showing the discontinuities on the top surface and corresponding spectra from EDX indicating the presence of Tungsten and Oxygen.

4.2 Thermal stability of W/B_4C multilayer mirrors

Multilayer mirrors used for space applications undergo a periodic temperature variation as the satellite orbits around the earth. The dynamic range and the profile of temperature variation depend on the orbital period and inclination. The orbital period of a satellite in a typical low earth orbit is around 90 minutes. The temperature of the ambiance varies from $+50^oC$ during sunlit position -40^oC during the earth occultation. Such a frequent and rapid temperature variation may result in the degradation in the performance of multilayer mirrors. This can be due to the rapid expansion and contraction of contrasting materials in the multilayer mirrors. Difference in the thermal expansion coefficients the W layer ($4.5 \times 10^{-6}/^oC$), B_4C layer ($5 \times 10^{-6}/^oC$) and the Si substrate ($2.6 \times 10^{-6}/^oC$) may results in the increase of interlayer roughness of the multilayer mirrors. In order to understand the effects of thermal cycling on W/B_4C multilayer structure, we have cycled several samples with various period and the number of bilayers for 1 day, 3 days and 10 days respectively. Different samples are used for different cycling periods. As these mirrors are known to have a significant change in their performance during their first few months after fabrication, all the samples chosen are at least one year old so as not to misinterpret the effect of thermal cycling with the longtime variations of the mirrors. Thermal cycling for all samples is done in air from $+55^oC$ to -40^oC at a rate of 2° per minute with a hold time of 15 minutes at the extreme temperatures. Figure 4.8 shows the thermal cycling profile which is applied to the mirrors.

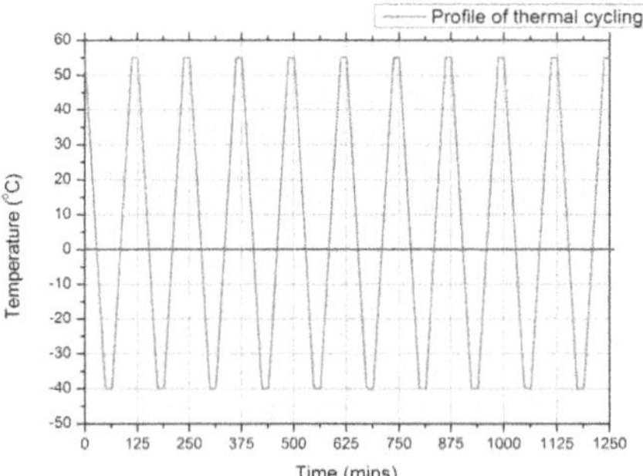

Figure 4.8: Profile of thermal cycling which is emulates the temperature profile of a satellite in a low earth orbit. W/B_4C multilayer mirrors of different specifications are subjected to this profile for 1, 3 and 10 days.

4.2.1   One-day thermal cycling

We have cycled four samples of W/B_4C multilayer mirrors of which two are of period 3.33 nm (d-3.3a, d-3.3b) and two are of period 5.2 nm and 5.4 nm respectively. Cycling is conducted for one day (20 cycles). Figure 4.9 and 4.10 shows the comparison of 8 keV reflectivity profile of four samples pre and post cycling. The reflectivity of all the samples remained mostly unchanged due to cycling. Peak reflectivities at first Bragg peak for all the samples before and after cycling are presented in table 4.2. It is observed that the thermal cycling for one day did not result in any significant changes in the structural parameters and performance of the mirrors. No trace of contamination layer formation is seen in these samples due to thermal cycling in air.

4.2.2   Three days thermal cycling

We have conducted continuous three days cycling (60 cycles) on the different set of samples. We have chosen three samples with periods 1.5 nm and 300 number of layer pairs (d-1.5), 4.4 nm (d-4.4), and 5.4 nm (d-5.4) with 50 layer pairs each. Figure 4.11 compares the reflectivity profiles of the sample d-1.5 at 8 keV lab source before and after thermal cycling for three days. It is observed that the peak reflectivity at the first Bragg peak remained mostly unchanged. However, we have observed a growth in the contamination layer thickness from 9.8 nm to 12.5 nm due to cycling. This can be due to an increase in oxidation of W layer over cycling in the air. As this sample is of the ultra-short period, the top B_4C layer is discontinuous which allows the bottom W layer to react with atmospheric

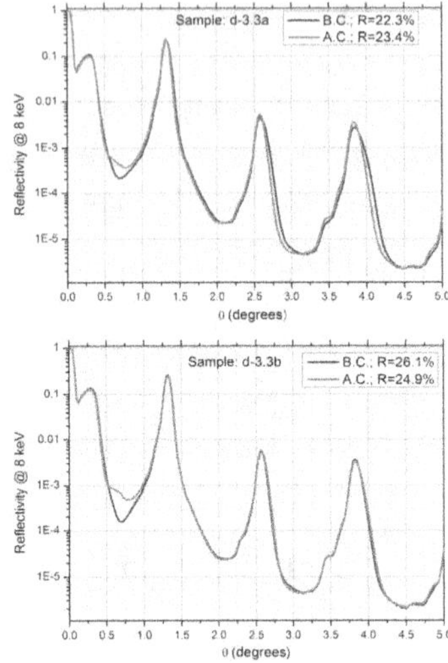

Figure 4.9: Comparison of reflectivity profiles of two samples with identical periods (d-3.3a and d-3.3b) with 70 number of bi-layers before and after one day cycling (20 thermal cycles).B.C. and A.C. in the inset represents before and after cycling data respectively.

oxygen to form a contamination layer. The double peak at the Bragg peak is due to Cu-kβ line coming directlyfrom the source.

Figure 4.12 and 4.13 compares the change in the reflectivity profile due to the three-day cycling of d-4.4 and d-5.4 samples respectively. There is little change in the reflectivity in the sample d-4.4 from 38.7% to 33.14% due to cycling. This can be due to a slight increase in interlayer roughness from 0.85 nm to 0.9 nm in the B_4C-W interface layers. Peak reflectivity of the sample d-5.4 is mostly unchanged over thermal cycling. In both the samples, the grazing incidence reflectivity profile between the critical angle cut-off and the first Bragg peak looks identical. This suggests that there is no sign of contamination layer formation on the top surface due to thermal cycling. Peak reflectivities at first Bragg peak for all the samples

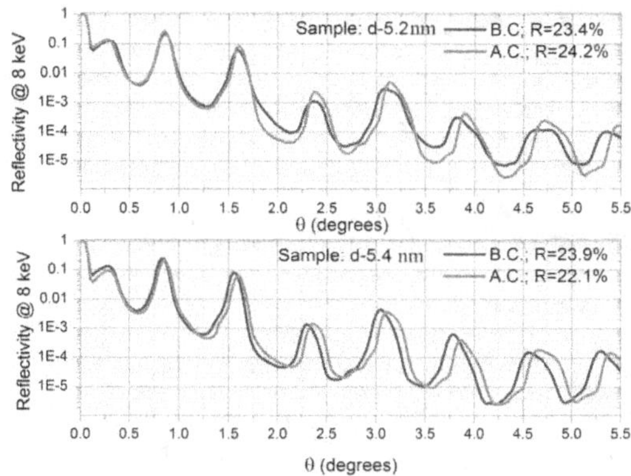

Figure 4.10: Comparison of reflectivity profiles of two samples with near equal periods (d-5.2 and d-5.4) with 50 number of bi-layers before and after one day cycling (20 thermal cycles).B.C. and A.C. in the inset represents before and after cycling data respectively.

before and after three-day thermal cycling are presented in table 4.2.

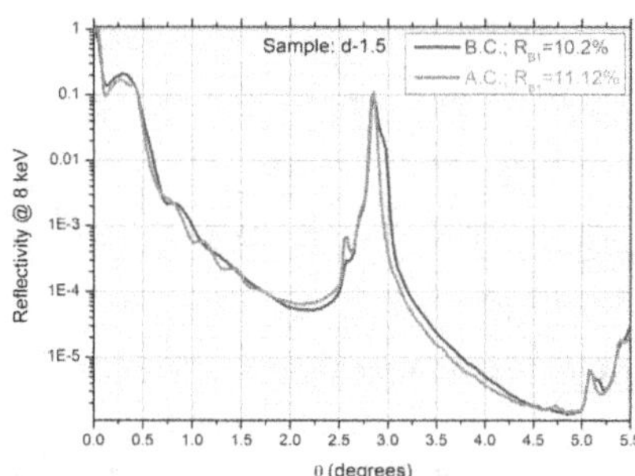

Figure 4.11: Comparison of reflectivity profiles of a W/B_4C multilayer mirror sample with period 1.5 nm and 300 layer pairs after three-day thermal cycling.

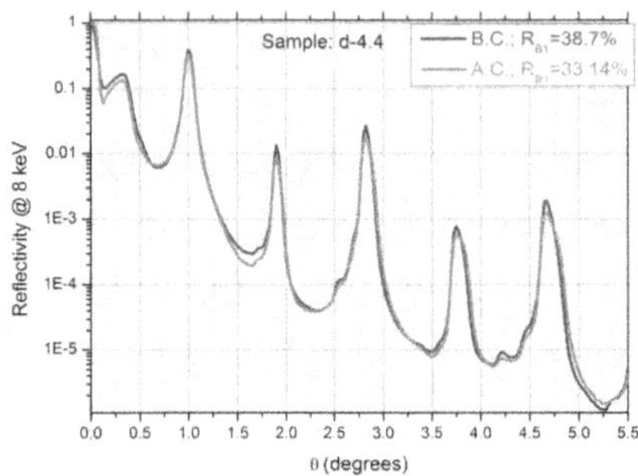

Figure 4.12: Comparison of reflectivity profiles of a W/B_4C multilayer mirror sample with period 4.4 nm and 50 layer pairs after three-day thermal cycling.

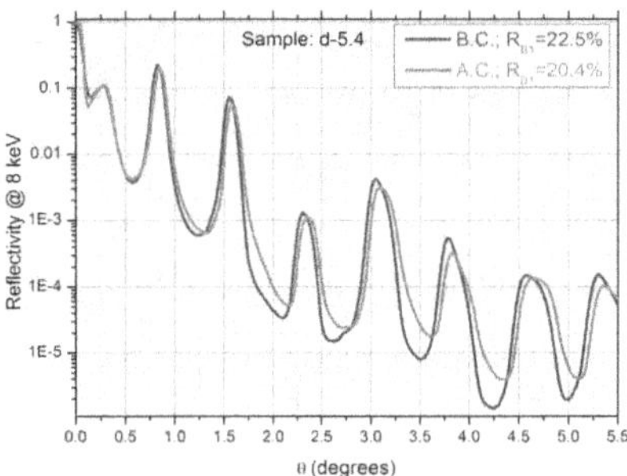

Figure 4.13: Comparison of reflectivity profiles of a W/B_4C multilayer mirror sample with period 5.4 nm and 50 layer pairs after three-day thermal cycling.

4.2.3 Ten-day thermal cycling

We have conducted long-term thermal cycling for ten days ($\sim$200 cycles) on two different samples with period 1.6 nm (d-1.6) and 3.2 nm (d-3.2). Figure 4.14 and 4.15 shows the comparison of reflectivity of profiles at 8 keV after ten day cycling for samples d-1.6 and d-3.2 respectively. Peak reflectivities of both the samples remained unchanged even after ten days of thermal cycling when measured at 8 keV. In the case of the d-1.5 sample, the contamination layer thickness is increased from 15 nm to 17.5 nm due to cycling. It is also observed that the roughness of the contamination layer is increased from 1 nm to 1.5 nm. The change in contamination layer thickness is similar to that in the case of three days cycling for a different sample with a similar period. From figure 4.15 it is observed for the sample d-3.2, the roughness in the contamination layer increased from 0.8 nm to 2 nm due to cycling. There is also a slight increase in the interlayer diffusion which can be seen from the profile between higher order Bragg peaks.

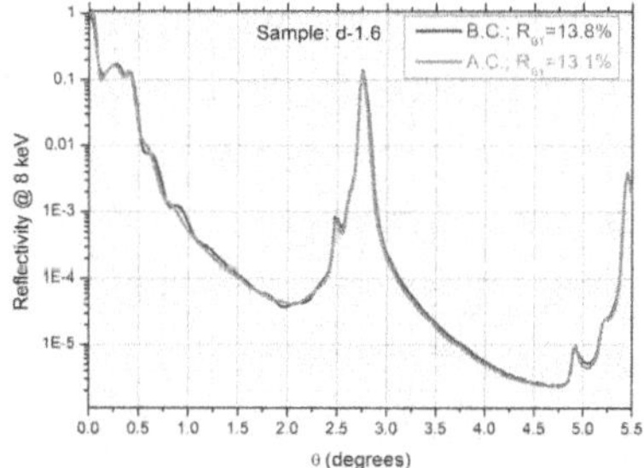

Figure 4.14: Comparison of reflectivity profiles of a W/B_4C multilayer mirror sample with period 1.6 nm and 300 layer pairs after ten-day thermal cycling.

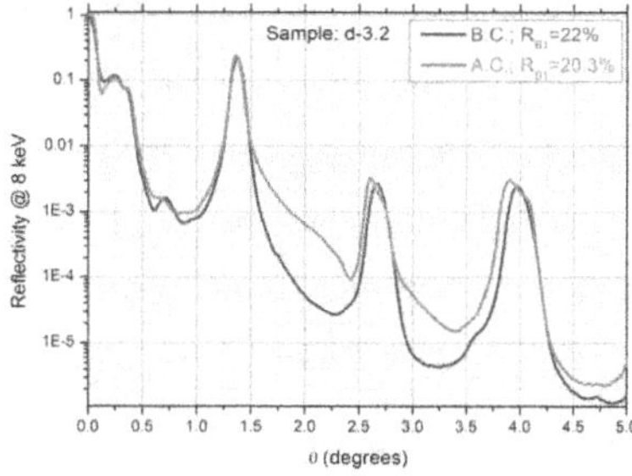

Figure 4.15: Comparison of reflectivity profiles of a W/B_4C multilayer mirror sample with period 3.2 nm and 50 layer pairs after ten-day thermal cycling.

Table 4.2: Comparisons of measured 1st order Bragg peak reflectivity at 8.047 keV of W/B_4C multilayer mirrors with varying periods.

Sample	R (before thermal cycling)	R (after thermal cycling)
	One-day thermal cycling	
d-3.3a	22.3 ±1.1	23.4 ±1.2
d-3.3b	26.1 ±1.5	24.9 ±1.5
d-5.2	23.4 ±1.2	24.2 ±1.5
d-5.4	23.9 ±1.4	22.1 ±1.3
	Three-day thermal cycling	
d-1.5	10.2 ±0.6	11.1 ±0.66
d-4.4	38.7 ±2.3	33.1 ±2
d-5.4	22.5 ±1.3	20.4 ±1.2
	Ten-day thermal cycling	
d-1.6	13.8 ±0.8	13.1 ±0.7
d-3.2	22 ±1.3	20.3 ±1.2

4.3 Soft X-ray reflectivity measurements

Major applications of constant period multilayer mirrors are in the soft X-ray region. Photon limited observations at X-ray energies from astrophysical sources demands maximum reflectivity from multilayer mirrors for polarimetric applications. W/B_4C multilayer mirrors have a good reflectivity and spectral resolution at soft X-ray region as these materials are free from absorption edges in this region [Jankowski et al., 1989], [Jankowski. et al., 1990], [Pradhan et al., 2018]. However many other material combinations are studied for wide energy range astrophysical applications [Windt et al., 2004]. Although most of the structural parameters of a multilayer mirror can be derived from HXR measurement, it is important to measure the optical performance at soft x-ray energies for the actual polarimetric applications. Also, it is observed that the structural parameters like roughness impact differently for hard X-ray and soft X-ray energies as they probe different roughness scales and spatial frequencies. In order to maintain high energy resolution, the FWHM (full width at half maximum) of Bragg peak (ΔE) should be minimized. We measured the energy resolution of multilayer mirrors using energy scans at soft X-rays in a synchrotron beamline. ΔE is small for mirrors with a large number of bi-layers (N).

A systematic pre- and post-thermal cycling SXR measurements were carried out to understand the effects of thermal cycling on the optical performance of multilayer mirrors. Three multilayer samples d-1.5, d-4.4 and d-5.4 were cycled for three days (same samples are used for HXR). Unlike the hard X-ray reflectivity results, a significant reduction in the measured reflectivity is observed at soft X-rays. There is no major change in ΔE of the multilayer mirrors at soft X-rays due to cycling. The growth of a contamination layer thickness in d-1.5 sample is also observed using SXR tests which is consistent with that derived from HXR results. Table 4.3 shows the comparison of pre- and post- thermal cycling 1st Bragg reflectivity and energy resolution of three multilayer samples at four different energies of 0.75 keV, 1 keV, 1.2 keV, and 1.5 keV.

Figure 4.16 shows measured data of both the angle-dependent SXR as well as the energy-dependent SXR around the 1st Bragg peak of all three samples, before and after thermal cycling. For sample d-1.5, interface oscillations are observed between the critical angle and the 1st Bragg peak in the angle-dependent SXR measured data. This indicates the presence of a contamination layer at the top of the multilayer film. The best-fit results indicate that thickness of the contamination layer increased from 10 nm to 11.4 nm with its interface width increasing from 1 nm to 1.25 nm after cycling. These values agree with measurements at hard X-rays. Unlike HXR measurements, there is a reduction in the measured peak reflectivity at soft X-rays. This suggests that the high-frequency spatial roughness of the mirror is unchanged whereas low-frequency spatial roughness increases after cycling. Hard X-rays probe high-frequency spatial roughness and as the wave-

Table 4.3: Soft X-ray reflectivity of multilayer mirrors with different periods measured before and after 3-day thermal cycling days (B.C- before thermal cycling, A.C. - after thermal cycling), Measured energy resolution ΔE in the units of eV at FWHM is given in bold. N = the number of layer pairs, of samples are listed.

Energy	0.75 keV	1 keV	1.2 keV	1.5 keV
d-1.5, N- 300				
R(B.C)	0.3 ±0.01	1.6 ±0.01	2.4 ±0.12	2.7 ±0.13
R(A.C)	0.2 ±0.01	1.9 ±0.01	2 ±0.1	2.5 ±0.12
ΔE (B.C)	-	12 ±1	15 ±1	21 ±2
ΔE (A.C)	-	19 ±1	16 ±1	22 ±2
d-44, N- 50				
R(B.C)	10.2 ±0.5	27.1 ±1.35	32.9 ±1.64	38.4 ±1.92
R(A.C)	5.2 ±0.26	17.3 ±0.01	23.2 ±1.16	27.5 ±1.37
ΔE (B.C)	-	50 ±3	47 ±3	67 ±
ΔE (A.C)	-	52 ±3	60 ±3	70 ±4
d-5.4b, N- 50				
R(B.C)	16.8 ±0.84	41.7 ±2.08	46.3 ±2.31	47.4 ±2.37
R(A.C)	7.4 ±0.37	29.7 ±1.48	33.9 ±1.69	37.4 ±1.87
ΔE (B.C)	-	49 ±3	73 ±4	88 ±4
ΔE (A.C)	-	57 ±3	65 ±4	74 ±4

length increases, the measurements are more sensitive to low spatial frequency roughness. Table 4.4 gives the structural parameters of the mirror obtained from fitting soft X-ray reflectivity data.

Figure 4.17 shows the comparison of the percentage change in the reflectivity of the 1st Bragg peaks at hard X-rays (8.047 keV) and soft X-rays (1.5 keV) for three different samples over three-day thermal cycling. The change in reflectivity is higher at soft X-rays than at hard X-rays. Thermal cycling results in an increase in the low-frequency roughness of W/B_4C multilayer mirrors while the high-frequency roughness remains mostly unchanged. It is also observed that the

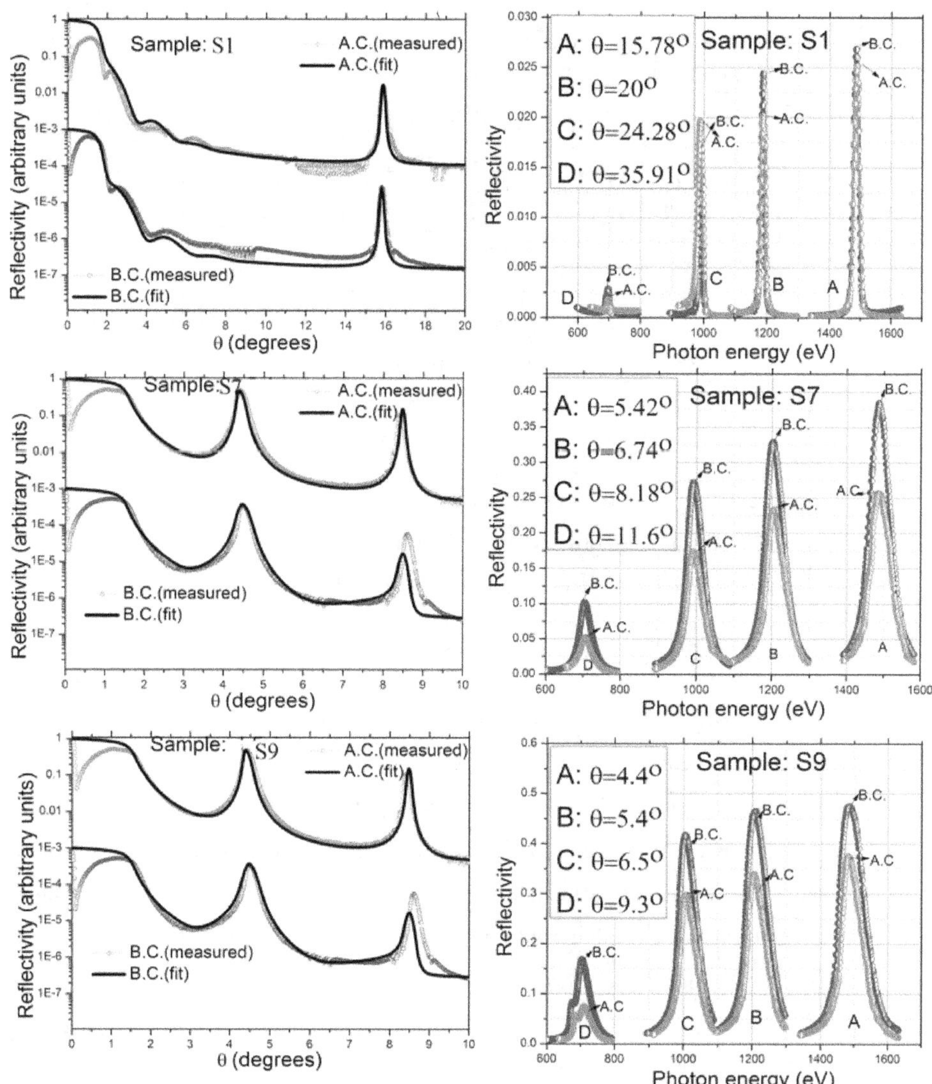

Figure 4.16: Measured angle dependent SXR at 1.5 keV (left side) and corresponding energy dependent SXR around the 1st Bragg peak in linear scale (right side) of three multilayer samples (top, d-1.5; middle, d-4.4; bottom, d-5.4). Before cycling and after cycling data is shown in blue and red respectively. Best fit model is given in black. Pre-cycling data and fit shown the left is offset by 10^{-3} for better clarity of the plot.

Table 4.4: The best-fit results for interface width of three multilayer mirrors obtained from angle dependent SXR at 1.5 keV.

Parameter	B_4C roughness (nm)	W roughness (nm)
	d-1.5, N- 300	
B.C	0.35 ±0.03	0.45 ±0.04
A.C	0.36 ±0.03	0.47 ±0.05
	d-44, N- 50	
B.C	0.37 ±0.04	0.48 ±0.05
A.C	0.55 ±0.05	0.69 ±0.07
	d-5.4b, N- 50	
B.C	0.37 ±0.04	0.41 ±0.04
A.C	0.6 ±0.06	0.68 ±0.07

low-frequency roughness increases for thicker bi-layers. This conclusion is partially confirmed from imaging observations of layer morphology of multilayer mirrors before and after thermal cycling using a Scanning Electron Microscope (SEM). No wrinkle formation is seen on the top of multilayer with a short period (d-4.4 and d-5.4) after the thermal cycling. As the period of multilayer increases, the formations of wrinkles become more evident. Figure 4.18 shows wrinkle patterns observed on multilayer samples. These features have dimensions of the order of a few tens of microns. This observation supports the argument of an increase in low spatial frequency roughness. Earlier studies have shown similar effects of wrinkle formation after heat treatment of depth-graded Pt/C multilayer mirrors [Maeda et al., 2015]. This wrinkle formation can be due to the compressive stress induced in the multilayer mirrors during cycling.

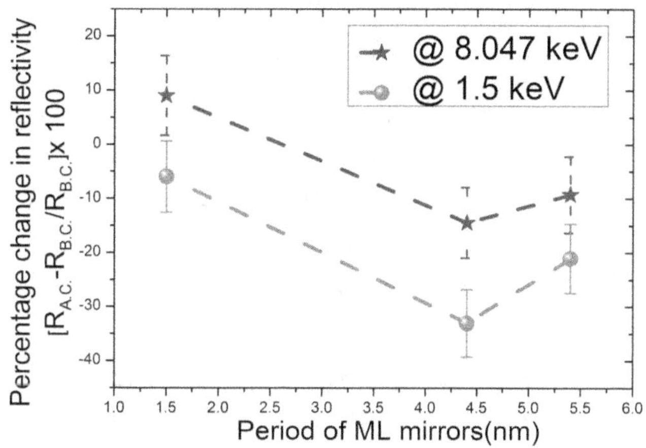

Figure 4.17: Comparison of percentage change in the reflectivity of the 1st Bragg peaks at hard X-rays (8.047 keV) and soft X-rays (1.5 keV) for three different samples after a 3-day thermal cycling.

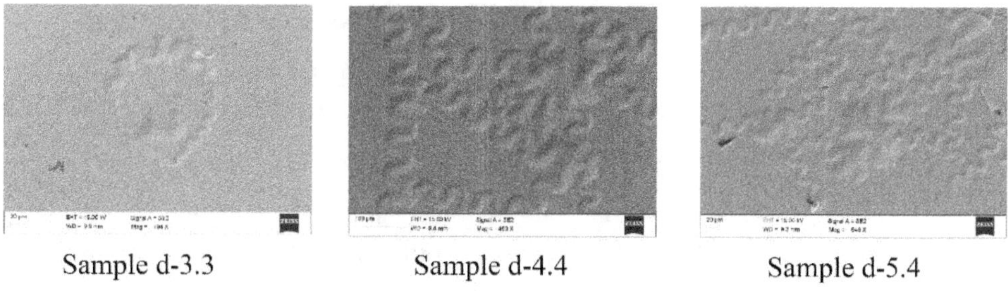

Sample d-3.3   Sample d-4.4   Sample d-5.4

Figure 4.18: Scanning electron microscopy analysis of the surface of three different samples after three-day thermal cycling.

4.4   Residual stress measurement of multilayer mirrors

Besides the reflective properties of the multilayer mirrors, the stability and imaging properties of mirrors also depend on the stress in the multilayer mirrors. $W/B4C$ multilayer mirrors can undergo thin film stress of the order of a few hundreds of megaPascals (MPa) [Jiang et al., 2015], [Majhi et al., 2018]. Such high stresses can deform the mirror and also results in the peeling off of the films from the substrate. Stress values significantly change by the fabrication process, size and shape of the substrate. Stress in thin films is classified into two types: Growth or Intrinsic stress and Induced or Extrinsic stress [Freund and Suresh, 2004]. Growth or intrinsic stress is introduced during the fabrication of the multilayer mirrors. Origin of this kind of stress can be due to the mismatch in the lattice parameters between two adjacent materials, the surface temperature during deposition, the rate of deposition, plasma pressure for sputtering, the formation of pores/islands during deposition, incorporation of impurities, the mobility of atoms, etc. Induced or extrinsic stress arise from the changes in the physical environment of the film material following the film deposition. Some of the reasons cause extrinsic stress are temperature change with a difference in coefficient of thermal expansions, electrostatic response to an electric field, chemical reactions between the different materials, bulk diffusion of layer etc.

Due to elastic properties of the film, the thin film stress induces the force on to the substrate which causes the bending of the mirror. Based on the type of curvature induced on the substrate by the film, the stress in the film is divided into two categories: Compressive stress (convex) and Tensile stress (concave). Compressive stress bends the substrate to make it more convex and the tensile stress makes it more concave. Figure 4.19 shows the schematic of mirror becoming convex of

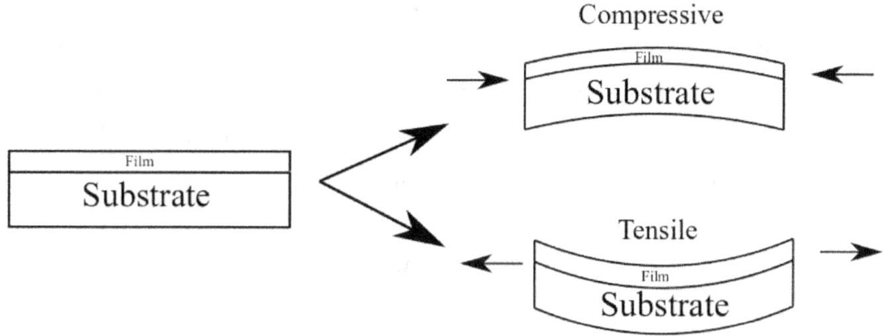

Figure 4.19: Schematic representing the effect of residual film stress on the substrate. An initial flat mirror will either becomes convex of concave depending on the type of stress induced by the film.

concave based on the type of residual stress. The nature of the stress depends on the film thickness, type of material, plasma pressure during deposition. Most materials initially form compressive stress for small thickness films and become tensile for intermediate thickness and again shows compressive stress for large thickness. Metallic films are usually more compressive than the dielectric layers. In a bilayer of a multilayer mirror, the compressive stress introduced by reflector (metallic) layer can be compensated by the tensile nature of spacer (dielectric) layer. Overall stress of a bilayer is given by the sum of both stresses induced on the layer. Compressive stress is usually represented as negative stress while the tensile stress is considered as positive stress.

4.4.1   Extrinsic thermal stress in W/B_4C multilayer mirror

Stress can be induced in a system due to change in ambient temperature of the mirror. This is mainly due difference in the thermal expansion between the substrate, reflector layer and the spacer layer. Thermal stress (Υ_t)is given by 4.1 [Freund and Suresh, 2004], [Thornton and Hoffman, 1989].

$$\Upsilon_t = \frac{E_f}{1 - V_f}\Delta\alpha(T_d - T_m) \tag{4.1}$$

where T_d and T_m are the ambient temperature during deposition and measurement respectively. E_f and v_f the Young's modulus and poisson's ratio of the film material. A great number of stress measurements in deposited layers are associated with the determination of the substrate curvature. Considering the small deviation in the curvature from almost flat substrate, the residual stress (Υ) in the thin film is best determined by Stoney's equation [Stoney, 1918].

$$\Upsilon = \frac{E_f}{1 - V_f}\frac{D^2}{6t}\left(\frac{1}{R_2} - \frac{1}{R1}\right) \tag{4.2}$$

where D is the substrate thickness, R_1 and R_2 are the radii of curvature of the mirror before and after coating, t is the total thickness of the film. Hence by measuring the radius of curvature of the mirror before and after coating one calculate the stress induced in the mirror due to fabrication. The stress induced due to induced/extrinsic reasons can be calculated by the precise measurement of change in radius of the sample.

We have measured the change in residual stress of W/B_4C multilayer mirrors due to one-day thermal cycling by measuring the radius of curvature of the mirrors both before and after thermal treatment. We thermal cycling four samples (d-3.3a, d-3.3b, d-5.2 and d-5.4) as described in table 4.2 for one-day thermal cycling. We have used the KLA Tencor system at IISc, mechanical engineering department to

Table 4.5: Summary of change in radius of curvature and residual stress of W/B_4C multilayer mirrors over one-day thermal cycling.

Sample	R_1 (B.C.) (m)	R_2 (A.C.) (m)	Change in ROC (m)	Change in stress (M Pa)
d-3.3a	-19.564	-20.726	-1.162	103.774
d-3.3b	-46.600	-49.962	-3.362	53.963
d-5.2	-16.977	-19.110	-2.133	194.174
d-5.4	-14.485	-17.700	-3.215	377.767

measure the radius of curvature. Initial radii of all mirrors are negative which indicates the compressive nature of the stress. The radius of curvature of all samples slightly reduced over one-day thermal cycling. This indicates that positive stress is induced in the mirrors due to thermal cycling. It is also observed large period multilayer mirrors are more affected to the thermal treatment. Table 4.5 presents the radius of curvature of the mirrors before and after measurements and also the change in residual stress in MPa calculated using Stoney's equation. As mentioned in section 4.2, there is no significant change in the reflectivity of the multilayer mirrors due to thermal cycling. However, over an extended period of thermal cycling (3-day cycling), we have observed a significant change in performance for large period multilayer mirrors. This clearly suggests that the large period multilayer are more sensitive to change in temperature of the surroundings.

4.5 Summary

The thermal cycling tests simulating the space environment in a typical low earth orbit, show small changes in the optical performance and structural properties of the W/B_4C multilayer mirrors. Earlier studies suggested that the period of W/B_4C multilayer mirrors change due to thermal annealing [Jankowski. et al.,

1990], [Rao et al., 2013]. But with thermal cycling within the above-mentioned range of temperatures, we have not observed any change in the period due to cycling. Changes in structural parameters of mirrors due to cycling are more sensitive to mirror performance at soft X-ray region than at hard X-ray energies. For the same samples, we observed that the SXR shows a reduction while the change in HXR is negligible. This suggests that the interlayer roughness/ diffusion increases at low spatial frequency scales while the high-frequency roughness/diffusion remains mostly unchanged. Further studies on the effect of thermal cycling on residual stress have to be carried out to understand the effect of wrinkle formation which will be a part of our future work. It is observed that short period (< 2 nm) multilayers are relatively more stable both structurally and in its optical performance over thermal cycling than large period (> 3 nm) multilayer mirrors. These findings are consistent with the stress analysis due to one-day thermal cycling. The change in residual stress in large period multilayer mirrors is significantly higher than the change in short period multilayer mirrors. Long-time performance evaluation of W/B_4C multilayer mirrors has indicated the formation of an oxidation layer on short period multilayer mirrors. However, the contamination layer thickness tends to saturate within a year after fabrication. Thermal cycling did not affect the energy resolution of multilayer mirrors in both hard X-ray and soft X-ray regions. For most astronomical applications, constant period multilayer mirrors are envisaged for operation only at the 1st Bragg peak condition. Hence slight variations in the grazing angle reflectivity and reflectivity at higher order Bragg peaks are not a major concern for these applications. From the above results, we conclude that constant period W/B_4C multilayer mirrors are suitable for space applications as they are nearly stable over time and minimally impacted over changing the thermal environment.

Chapter 5

Soft X-ray polarimetry

5.1 Polarization of an electromagnetic wave

The polarization of photons is the fundamental nature of electromagnetic waves. A photon is a discrete packet of time-varying electric and magnetic fields oriented transverse to the direction of propagation. The polarization describes the configuration of these fields. This configuration explains the physical processes that emits a particular photon. Since electric and magnetic fields are interrelated through Maxwell's equations, the configurations of both fields are set by the specification of the electric field alone.

An electromagnetic plane wave propagating along the z-axis with angular frequency ω can be described as a sinusoidally varying electric field of the form (5.1),

$$\bar{E} = \hat{x}E_X + \hat{y}E_Y = \hat{x}E_{oX}cos(kz - \omega t) + \hat{y}E_{oY}cos(kz - \omega t + \varepsilon) \qquad (5.1)$$

where,

ε is the ratio of E_{oX} and E_{oY},

E_{oX} and E_{oY} are amplitudes of electric fields along x and y directions respectively,

$\hat{x}$ and $\hat{y}$ are unit vectors along x and y directions respectively,

$k = \omega/c$.

Polarization is symmetric about 180° rotation. The wave is linearly polarized when E_X and E_Y are proportional. From equation (5.1), this occurs when $\varepsilon = n\pi$ where 'n' is an integer.If $\varepsilon \neq n\pi$, the electric field rotates as a function of time or position, which is termed elliptical polarization. Polarization is further classified as left and right according to whether $\bar{E}$ rotates clockwise or anti-clockwise respectively. Circular polarization is a special case of elliptical polarization where $E_{oX} = E_{oY}$. The polarization angle of linear polarization is given by $tan^{-1}\left(\frac{E_{0X}}{E_{oY}}\right)$.

Each individual photon has a defined state of polarization. However, multiple photons from the same source may have different polarizations. If polarization states of all photons are not random, then the source has a net non zero polarization. The Stokes parameters [Stokes, 1851] provide a means to fully characterize the polarization of a source using four parameters ((5.2) to (5.5)):

$$I = \langle E_{oX}^2 \rangle + \langle E_{oY}^2 \rangle \tag{5.2}$$

$$Q = \langle E_{oX}^2 \rangle - \langle E_{oY}^2 \rangle \tag{5.3}$$

$$U = \langle 2E_{oX}E_{oY}\cos\varepsilon \rangle \tag{5.4}$$

$$V = \langle 2E_{oX}E_{oY}\sin\varepsilon \rangle \tag{5.5}$$

From above equations, I gives the information about total intensity of the light, Q describes linear horizontal or vertical polarization, U describes linear polarization at 45° and V gives information about circularly polarized component of the light. These are calculated as averages over multiple photons detected from the source.

5.2 Techniques for measuring X-ray polarimetry

Available X-ray detectors are able to measure the intensity, energy and the position at which X-rays deposit charge via interactions but not polarization state directly. Hence X-rays must undergo some interactions that translate polarization information into any of the above three mentioned parameters which detectors can detect (usually intensity). There are only a limited number of ways to measure the linear polarization of X-rays in 0.1-50 keV band. The difficulty is mainly due to the lack of many elements that can efficiently interact with the polarization property of the X-ray. An important concern which makes x-ray polarimetry very difficult is that the modulation factor of polarization analyzers is very low (20% to 40%) with an exception for Bragg-crystal polarimeter. Also, most astronomical sources are not expected to emit strongly polarized x-rays ($\gg 10\%$) which further reduces the probability of having confident observations.

In-spite of above mentioned difficulties, some techniques are available that promise to reveal the polarization state of x-rays that sheds light on the physical processes in the source. Different fundamental processes dominate the interaction of photons at different photon energies. Photoelectric interactions dominate at low energies, Compton scattering dominates at intermediate energies and pair production dominates at high energies of the electromagnetic spectrum.

Pair production technique is dominant in gamma ray region and extreme hard x-rays. Popular techniques used for x-ray polarimetry are as follows:

- Bragg reflection polarimeters for soft X-rays (0.1 to 5 keV).

- Photoelectric X-ray polarimeters for soft X-rays (2 to 10 keV).

- Compton/Thomson scattering polarimeters for hard X-rays ($\sim$ 20 to 200 keV)

5.2.1 Compton/ Thompson scattering polarimeter

Compton scattering [Compton, 1923] is the dominant process at energies above a few tens of keV. When X-rays with sufficient energy interact with the matter, the electrons will recoil, taking the energy from the photon. At low energy X-rays, the recoil of the electron is negligible which limits the case to Thompson scattering. The differential cross-section for Compton scattering of X-rays is given by Klein-Nishina formula [Heitler, 1954] (5.6),

$$\frac{d\sigma}{d\Omega} = \frac{r_e^2}{2}\left(\frac{E'}{E}\right)^2\left(\frac{E'}{E} + \frac{E}{E'} - 2sin^2\theta cos^2\phi\right) \tag{5.6}$$

where r_e is the classical radius of an electron, E is the initial photon energy, E' is the final photon energy after scattering. The initial and final photon energies varies as a function of scattering angle "θ" as (5.7),

$$E' = E\left[1 + (1 - cos\theta)\frac{E}{m_e c^2}\right]^{-1} \tag{5.7}$$

For scattering angles close to 90°, the azimuthal distribution of the scattered photon is strongly dependent on the polarization state of the incident photon. Hence by measuring the azimuthal distribution of the scattered photons, one can measure the polarization state of the incident photon.

Figure 5.1 shows the schematic of the functioning of basic Compton/Thompson scattering polarimeters. X-rays from the source get scattered from the target to a detector. The target-detector is typically arranged at 90° to maximize the scattering-detection efficiency of the set-up. A detector then records the azimuthal distribution of the scattered photons which contains the information of degree of polarization and angle of the incident X-rays. An ideal event is the one in which the photon scatters once in a scattering element and is subsequently absorbed by the X-ray detector. Compton scattering does not require a distinction between scatterer and a detector hence it can be observed in an array of detectors. However, the sensitivity of polarization detection can be improved by using a low Z scatterer as it will increase the efficiency of Compton scattering and reduces the photoelectric absorption of the scattered X-rays inside the target. Use of low Z scatter has a disadvantage of poor energy resolution.

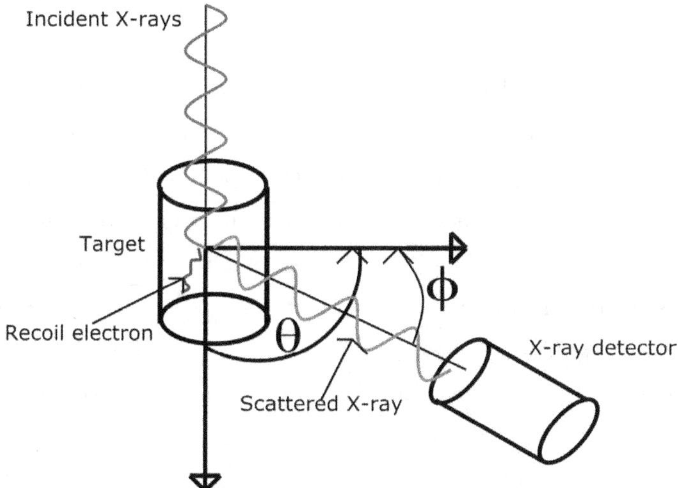

Figure 5.1: Schematic describing the function of a basic Compton/Thompson scattering polarimeter

For the best performance of the instrument the length of the target should be as large as possible to increase the number of interactions for Compton scattering and the diameter of the target should be kept as low as possible to reduce the photoelectric absorption of the scattered X-rays inside the target material. However as the thickness of the target reduces, effective photon collecting area of the instrument also comes down which reduces the overall sensitivity of the instrument. A hard X-ray focusing optics set-up in-front the target helps to increase the collection area of the instrument while keeping the thickness of the target.

First dedicated extra-solar X-ray polarimeter was a Thompson scattering polarimeter flown on a sounding rocket in 1969 [Angel et al., 1969]. Currently, many groups have been working on repeating this heritage. Most of the instruments have a low Z scatter surrounded by a series of X-ray detectors around it for recording azimuthal scattering information. The Gamma-Ray Burst polarimeter (GAP) was flown on-board Japanese IKAROS mission is a Compton scattering polarimeter operated in 50-300 keV band [Yonetoku et al., 2011]. CZT detector on-board the Indian mission Astrosat uses an array of Cadmium Zinc Tellurium detectors observed the Hard X-ray polarization degree and angle from Crab nebula [Vadawale et al., 2018]. CZT is originally designed as an imaging instrument. However, above 100 keV the collimator of the detectors become transparent and can measure the azimuthal distribution of the Compton scattering from the neighbouring pixels. A light-weight Polarised Gamma-ray Observer (PoGO+), balloon based Compton polarimeter has used the same technique and measured the polarization from the Crab Nebula at Hard X-ray region [Chauvin et al., 2018]. With the recent success of NuSTAR [Harrison and NuSTAR Science Team, 2004] mission demonstrating the focusing hard X-ray optics, new Compton polarimeters missions like PolSTAR [Krawczynski et al., 2016] uses a hard X-ray optics at front-end to increase the effective area and reduce the background of the instrument.

5.2.2 Photo electric polarimeter

In 1926, Auger discovered from his cloud chamber experiments that the direction of emitted photo electron depends on the linear polarization state of the incident X-ray photons [Auger, 1926]. The expression for the differential cross section distribution of the photoelectric effect, in the non-relativistic approximation, is given by (5.8)

$$\frac{\partial \sigma}{\partial \Omega} = r_o^2 \left(\frac{Z^5}{137^4} \right)^{7/2} \frac{4\sqrt{2}sin^2(\theta)cos^2(\varphi)}{(1 - \beta cos(\theta))^4} \tag{5.8}$$

where,

θ is polar angle between the direction of incoming photon and the ejected electron,

ψ azimuth angle of the ejected electron with respect to X-ray polarization vector,

Z is the atomic number of absorption material,

r_o classical radius of the electron,

β speed of electron in the units of c (velocity of light).

The sensitivity of the polarimeter is highest when scattering angle, $\theta = 90^o$ and reduces as the angle deviates from it. The photoelectron is preferentially emitted parallel to the photon electric field, i.e. the distribution peaks at $\theta = 90^o$. Once the photoelectron is emitted it leaves a trail of electron-ion pairs marking its path from the initial ejected electron to a final stopping point. Thus it is possible to measure the linear polarization of incident X-rays by measuring the initial direction of the ejected electron. The probability of ejecting a photoelectron perpendicular to the electric field vector is zero for an ideal polarization analyser. The major difficulty in this technique is that, when electrons interact with the matter, they give up most of the energy when velocities decrease towards the end of their track, not at the beginning. In the process of giving energy to the local medium, the electron may change its trajectory leading to loss of information about the polarization of X-rays. So, the complexity arises due to contradictory requirements of having high-efficiency material for converting the incident X-ray flux into photoelectrons and in restricting those photoelectrons to travel large distance before interacting with elements of the absorbing materials. Gas based detectors usually have larger path lengths which make it practically possible to track the electron path. In semiconductor detectors, the path length of the electron is very small, which makes it very difficult to track the initial and final direction. In silicon, the average path length of an electron produced by a 1 keV photon is 0.03 microns, while that for a 10 keV photon is 1 micron. But the minimum size of a silicon-based detector is 10 microns. This keeps the practical limitation of using a silicon based detector polarization measurement in this technique. In contrast, electron track length in neon at 1 atm and 0 C is 0.08 mm for 1 keV and 3 mm for 10 keV photon. Current gas-based detectors are available with a positional accuracy of 100 microns which makes it feasible to use a gas detector.

The key aspect of this technique is to track the photo-electron path in the detector. The electrons in the track must be channelled to readout electrodes at the edge of the detector. Electrons can be drifted through the gas by application of a uniform electric field. There are two possible configurations in which this drifting can be done (figure 5.2): Drift field across the direction of the incident photon (Costa geometry, [Costa et al., 2001]) and drift field along the perpendicular to the incident photon (Black geometry, [Black et al., 2007]). As the secondary electrons drift, they scatter on the gas atoms inside the detector material. This leads to the diffusion of electrons as they drift. This diffusion degrades the track image which reduces the modulation factor of the instrument. Imaging X-ray polarimetric explorer (IXPE) [Weisskopf et al., 2016], a dedicated X-ray polarimetric NASA's mission is under development which uses Costa's geometry detector for polarization measurement from 2-10 keV.

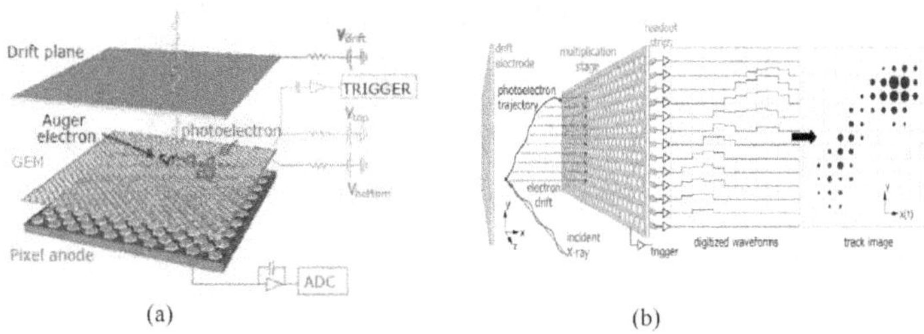

Figure 5.2: (a) Photoelectric polarimeter with Costa geometry. (b)Photoelectric polarimeter of Black geometry. Image courtesy: [Costa et al., 2001] and [Black et al., 2007]

Bragg reflection polarimeter

A flat crystal or multilayer mirror oriented at 45° to parallel X-rays acts as a perfect polarization analyzer of X-rays when Bragg's condition is satisfied. This is because the Brewster angle at X-ray region is at 45° for almost all material as the refractive index of all materials is very close to 1. At Brewster angle, when unpolarized light (a mixture of all polarization states of light) is incident on to a metallic surface, only S-polarized light is reflected but not P-polarized light. If input light is P-polarized, then the reflection is almost zero and when input light is S-polarized, then the reflection is maximum. Exploiting this condition of "polarization by reflection", an atomic crystal or a multilayer mirror can be used as a polarization analyzer. Though at soft X-rays, scattering is not a dominant process, superposition of coherent scattered X-rays from a periodic medium such as an atomic crystal or a multilayer mirror, can produce an efficient reflection.

The most successful measurement of cosmic X-ray polarization has been made with Bragg crystal polarimeters. X-ray polarimeter on OSO-8 satellite used graphite crystals with a mosaic spread of 0.8^o and an effective width of 3 eV. The instrument is rotated with a nominal frequency of 6 rpm and the signature of polarization is observed at twice the frequency. Using this polarimeter, modulation curve of Crab nebula is obtained at 2.6 keV which indicated that the polarization is 19.22% $\pm0.92\%$ and the angle of polarization is 155.770 ± 1.3^o [Weisskopf et al., 1978]. This was the first and only high precision X-ray polarization measurement obtained for any cosmic source and was in excellent agreement with optical polarization measurements of the Crab nebula.

Due to current development in the multilayer mirror fabrication technology, multilayer mirror based soft X-ray polarimeters are becoming popular. These are best suited for operation under 1 keV where other polarimetry techniques are less efficient and natural atomic Bragg crystals are not available. The polarimeter for Low Energy X-ray Astronomical Sources (PLEXAS) [Marshall et al., 1998] concept used a parabolic geometry similar to that of OSO-8 but with a Bragg energy near 250 eV. Other proposed instruments like Light Asymmetry and Magnetic Probe (LAMP) [She et al., 2015] uses the similar design of PLEXAS operating at 250 eV. The major disadvantage of Bragg crystal polarimetry is its narrow bandwidth which makes the instrument not optimal for braod-band spectroscopic studies for the scientific community.

New technologies like depth graded and laterally graded multilayer mirrors made it possible to develop broad band soft X-ray polarimeter under 1 keV. Rocket Experiment Demonstration of a Soft X-ray polarimeter (REDSoX polarimeter) [Marshall, 2015] has been proposed using the combination of CAT

(Critical Angle Transmission) grating [Heilmann et al., 2009] and laterally graded multilayer mirrors. This design is capable of measuring high-resolution spectro-polarimetric studies at soft X-rays ($< 1keV$).

5.3   Analyzing the polarization data

A polarimeter gives the data of intensity versus azimuthal angle. Figure 5.3 shows the setup of typical rotating linear polarization analyzer. The analyzer is rotated, the associated detector records the intensity of photons at each analyzer angle. The resultant histogram of counts versus rotation angle (modulation curve), is shown in figure 5.4 (for polarized a source).

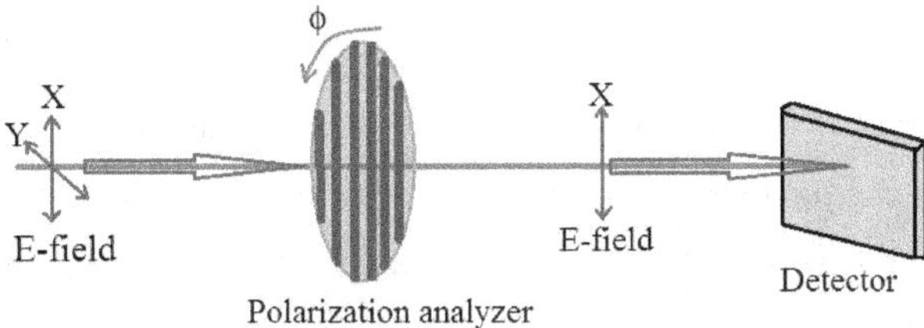

Figure 5.3: Schematic of a working of a basic polarimeter. Linear polarization analyzer is rotated and the detector records the intensity of photons as a function of the rotation angle of the analyzer.

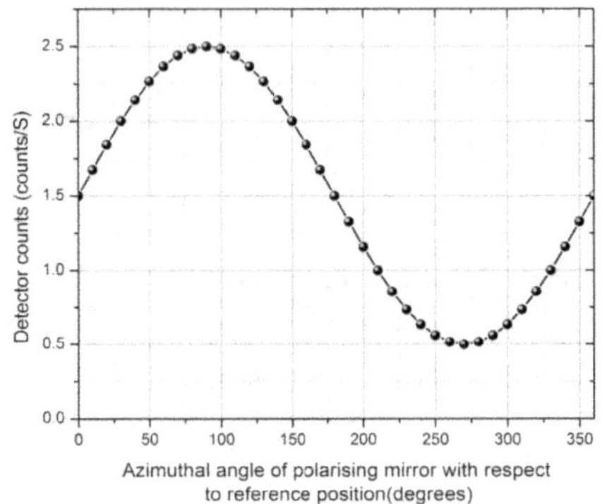

Figure 5.4: Typical modulation curve obtained by rotating the analyzer for a polarized source. (Units of y-axis are arbitrary)

General modulation curve as shown in the figure 5.4 will have the form (5.9),

$$S(\phi) = A + Bcos^2(\phi - \phi_o)$$
(5.9)

The polarization angle ϕ_o is the angle at which maximum intensity is recorded. 'A' describes the unpolarized component of the input intensity and 'B' describes the polarized intensity. ϕ is the rotational angle of the polarization analyzer. The modulation amplitude is given by, (5.10)

$$a = \frac{S_{max} - S_{min}}{S_{max} + S_{min}}$$
(5.10)

The modulation curve can also be written in terms of the Stoke's parameters as, (5.11)

$$S(\phi) = I + Qcos(2\phi) + Usin(2\phi)$$
(5.11)

Polarization analyzer of this type is not sensitive to circular polarization. Hence it is independent of V Stoke's parameter. Determining the Stokes's parameters is equivalent to measuring the source intensity in three different filters: Unpolarized, polarized at 0° and polarized at 45°. The Stokes parameters can be obtained directly from the modulation curve, (5.12)

$$I = \langle S(\phi) \rangle, Q = S(0^o) - I, U + I = S(45^o). \tag{5.12}$$

Another important parameter for a polarimeter is "modulation index (μ)". The modulation index of a polarimeter is defined as the modulation amplitude obtained by the instrument for a 100% polarized source. For an ideal polarimeter, the modulation index is 1. The most standard way of obtaining the percentage of polarization (P) and polarization angle (ψ) is by using Stokes parameters(I, Q, U). Two methods that directly calculates Stokes parameters from the modulation curve are discussed in this section.

5.3.1 Muller matrix approach

For a setup like Bragg reflection polarimeter, output Stokes vectors are obtained by pre-multiplying Muller matrix of the instrument to the Stokes parameters of the input light. In practice, output Stokes I vector, say, 'S_1' (total intensity) is measured from the detector. So, if the Muller matrix of the instrument is known, the relation between output Stokes I, S_1 and input stokes parameters (I,Q,U) can be obtained. Bragg reflection polarization analyzer is a linear polarizer with its transmission along x-axis and perpendicular axis along the y-axis. Let p_x and p_y are the reflection efficiencies along x and y-axis respectively. Since at Brewster angle, mirror or crystal behaves as a linear polarizer, its Muller matrix is given by,

(5.13)

$$M_p = 0.5 \times \begin{bmatrix} p_x^2 + p_y^2 & p_x^2 - p_y^2 & 0 & 0 \\ p_x^2 - p_y^2 & p_x^2 + p_y^2 & 0 & 0 \\ 0 & 0 & 2p_x p_y & 0 \\ 0 & 0 & 0 & 2p_x p_y \end{bmatrix} \tag{5.13}$$

Modulation curve is obtained by rotating the polarizer around its axis. Hence the Muller matrix of the system is obtained by post-multiplying the rotation Muller matrix to the Muller matrix of the polarizer. Muller matrix of a rotating element after a rotation of angle θ is given by, (5.13)

$$M_r = \begin{bmatrix} 1 & 0 & 0 & 0 \\ 0 & cos(2\theta) & sin(2\theta) & 0 \\ 0 & -sin(2\theta) & cos(2\theta) & 0 \\ 0 & 0 & 0 & 0 \end{bmatrix} \tag{5.14}$$

Muller matrix of the output is light is given by, (5.15)

$$S_{o(4\times1)} = M_{p(4\times4)} . M_{r(4\times4)} . S_i \tag{5.15}$$

Here S_i is the Stokes vectors of input light and S_o is the Stokes vector of output light observed at the detector. Solving above equation we get,

$$
\begin{bmatrix} S_1 \\ S_2 \\ S_3 \\ S_4 \end{bmatrix}
= 0.5 \times
\begin{bmatrix}
p_x^2 + p_y^2 & p_x^2 - p_y^2 & 0 & 0 \\
p_x^2 - p_y^2 & p_x^2 + p_y^2 & 0 & 0 \\
0 & 0 & 2p_x p_y & 0 \\
0 & 0 & 0 & 2p_x p_y
\end{bmatrix}
\times
\begin{bmatrix}
1 & 0 & 0 & 0 \\
0 & cos(2\theta) & sin(2\theta) & 0 \\
0 & -sin(2\theta) & cos(2\theta) & 0 \\
0 & 0 & 0 & 0
\end{bmatrix}
\times
\begin{bmatrix} I \\ Q \\ U \\ V \end{bmatrix}
$$

$$
= 0.5 \times
\begin{bmatrix}
p_x^2 + p_y^2 & (p_x^2 - p_y^2)cos(2\theta) & (p_x^2 - p_y^2)sin(2\theta) & 0 \\
p_x^2 - p_y^2 & (p_x^2 + p_y^2)cos(2\theta) & (p_x^2 + p_y^2)sin(2\theta) & 0 \\
0 & -(2p_x p_y)sin(2\theta) & (2p_x p_y)cos(2\theta) & 0 \\
0 & 0 & 0 & 2p_x p_y
\end{bmatrix}
\times
\begin{bmatrix} I \\ Q \\ U \\ V \end{bmatrix}
$$

Above equations can be written in equation form as, (5.16) to (5.19)

$$
S_1 = \frac{p_x^2 + p_y^2}{2}\,I + \frac{p_x^2 - p_y^2}{2}cos(2\theta)\,Q + \frac{p_x^2 - p_y^2}{2}sin(2\theta)\,U \qquad (5.16)
$$

$$
S_2 = \frac{p_x^2 - p_y^2}{2}\,I + \frac{p_x^2 + p_y^2}{2}cos(2\theta)\,Q + \frac{p_x^2 + p_y^2}{2}sin(2\theta)\,U \qquad (5.17)
$$

$$
S_3 = -p_x p_y sin(2\theta)\,Q + p_x p_y cos(2\theta)\,U \qquad (5.18)
$$

$$
S_4 = p_x p_y\,V \qquad (5.19)
$$

As the X-ray detectors are not sensitive to any polarization information of the incident beam, it measures only S_1 of the incident beam. Hence by observing the intensity at any three different azimuth angles, we can find the values of I, Q and U vectors. Since above equations are not a function V, one cannot measure the V vector of Stokes parameters (circular polarization). Hence once the modulation curve is obtained with any three points say (θ= 0,45 and 90) Stokes parameters of the input beam can be derived by, (5.20) to (5.22)

$$S_1(0) = \frac{p_x^2 + p_y^2}{2} I + \frac{p_x^2 - p_y^2}{2} Q \tag{5.20}$$

$$S_1(45) = \frac{p_x^2 + p_y^2}{2} I + \frac{p_x^2 - p_y^2}{2} U \tag{5.21}$$

$$S_1(90) = \frac{p_x^2 + p_y^2}{2} I - \frac{p_x^2 - p_y^2}{2} Q \tag{5.22}$$

By solving above three equations, Stokes parameters of input X-rays can be found out by, (5.23) to (5.25)

$$I = \frac{S_1(0) + S_1(90)}{p_x^2 + p_y^2} \tag{5.23}$$

$$Q = \frac{S_1(0) - S_1(90)}{p_x^2 - p_y^2} \tag{5.24}$$

$$U = \frac{2}{p_x^2 - p_y^2} S_1(45) - \frac{p_x^2 + p_y^2}{p_x^2 - p_y^2} I \tag{5.25}$$

For an ideal linear horizontal polarization analyzer, $p_x = 1$ and $p_y = 0$. Then the above equations is simplified to, (5.26) to (5.28)

$$I = S_1(0) + S_1(90) \tag{5.26}$$

$$Q = S_1(0) - S_1(90) \tag{5.27}$$

$$U = 2S_1(45) - I \tag{5.28}$$

5.3.2 Fitting the modulation curve

Modulation curve shown in figure 5.4 can be mathematically described as, (5.29)

$$S(\theta) = 0.5 \times (I + Q cos(2\theta) + U sin(2\theta)) \tag{5.29}$$

Since intensity cannot be negative and is a mix of unmodulated and modulated terms, the above equation can also be written in its general forms as, (5.30)

$$S(\theta) = A + B cos^2(\theta - C)$$

(5.30)

Equating above two equations, we get, (5.31) to (5.33)

$$I = 2A + B$$

(5.31)

$$Q = B\ cos(2C)$$

(5.32)

$$U = B\ sin(2C)$$

(5.33)

A, B and C are obtained by fitting the measured modulation curve with the function as mentioned in equation (5.31). Above equations assumes that the polarization analyzer is an ideal one i.e. p_x=1 and p_y=0. But in the case of practical polarization analyzers, the more general form is given by, (5.34) to (5.36)

$$I = \frac{2A + B}{(p_x^2 + p_y^2)}$$

(5.34)

$$Q = \frac{B\ cos(2C)}{(p_x^2 - p_y^2)}$$

(5.35)

$$U = \frac{B\ sin(2C)}{(p_x^2 - p_y^2)}$$

(5.36)

5.3.3   Polarization fraction and angle

Stokes parameters can be determined from either of the above-mentioned methods. Polarization fraction of the incident beam and the polarization angle can be calculated using Stokes parameters as, (5.37) and (5.38)

$$P = \frac{\sqrt{Q^2 + U^2}}{I} \tag{5.37}$$

$$\psi = 0.5 \times tan^{-1}\left(\frac{U}{Q}\right) \tag{5.38}$$

5.3.4 Figure of merit of the Instrument

In an X-ray polarimeter, the ability to make a significant observation of the system depends on the modulation factor, the number of photons received, and the amount of polarized or unpolarized background photons seen from the detector. In the presence of noise which follows Poison's distribution and if N is the total number of counts, the probability $p(a,\psi)$ of measuring a particular modulation amplitude a and phase ψ, given true amplitude and phase are a_o and ψ_o, is given by [Weisskopf et al., 2010], (5.39)

$$p(a, \psi) = \frac{Na}{4\pi} \; exp\left[-\frac{N}{4}[a^2 + a_o^2 - 2aa_o \; cos(\psi - \psi_o]\right] \tag{5.39}$$

a_o is equal to zero if the source is completely unpolarized. Since the modulation factor is a non-negative number, there is always a non-zero probability to measure amplitude modulation even for an unpolarized source. Figure 5.5 shows the probability of detecting a modulation amplitude of a source with true source modulation amplitude 0.5 and true and observed phase as 45° for different observations with different observed source counts. Figure 5.6 shows the probability of detecting polarization angle ψ given the true $\psi = 45^o$ and the true and observed modulation amplitude is equal to 1. It is observed that as the number of counts of observation increases, the confidence level of observation increases.

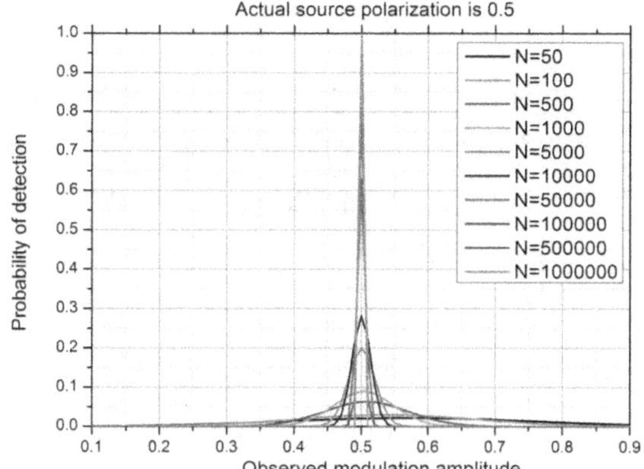

Figure 5.5: Probability of observing the modulation amplitude of the source with true modulation amplitude of 0.5 and observed and rue phase of the source is 45° for different observations with different source counts 'N'. As N increases, the confidence of observation increases. For small source counts, there an over estimation of the modulation amplitude

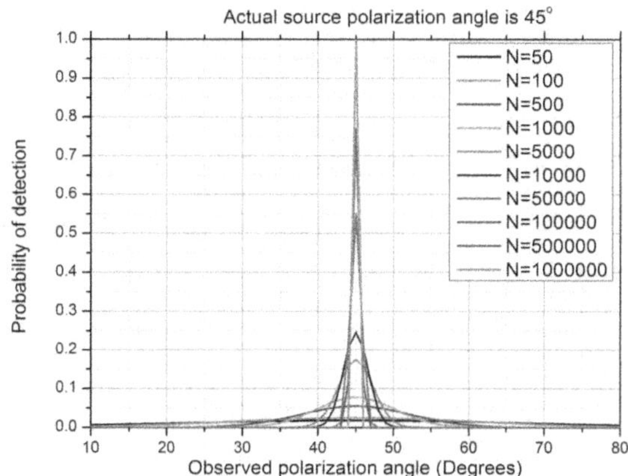

Figure 5.6: :Probability of detecting polarization angle ψ given the true $\psi = 45^o$ and the true and observed modulation amplitude is equal to 1 for different observations with different source counts.

Equation (5.39) can be used determine the amplitude which has a given probability of being exceeded by chance for an unpolarized source. For example the amplitude $a_{1\%}$, that has only 1% probability of being exceeded by chance is given by [Weisskopf et al., 2010], (5.40)

$$a_{1\%} = \frac{4.29}{\sqrt{N}} \tag{5.40}$$

In above equation N includes both source and background counts. Hence to express modulation amplitude as a function of detected signal alone, (5.41)

$$a_s = a_{1\%} \times \frac{R_s + R_b}{R_s} \tag{5.41}$$

Here R_s and R_b are the signal and background counting rates. Equation (5.41) gives the minimum detectable polarization of any source with 99% confidence level for those counts received given the instrument is an ideal polarization analyser i.e. μ of the instrument is equal to 1. But in practice, modulation index $\mu \leq 1$ and depends on the type of interaction of polarimeter and also on the energy of the photon. Considering the modulation index of the instrument the minimum detectable polarization (MDP) with 99% confidence or with 1% chance of exceeding the actual value is defined as [Weisskopf et al., 2010], (5.42)

$$MDP = \frac{a_s}{\mu} = \frac{4.29}{\mu R_s} \left[\frac{R_s + R_b}{T} \right]^{\frac{1}{2}} \tag{5.42}$$

T is the total duration of that particular observation. MDP is the traditional figure of merit for the X-ray polarimeter. However, MDP corresponds to detection of the amplitude of modulation that has only 1% probability of detection by chance but not the uncertainty of polarization measurement. If C ($0 \leq C \leq 1$) is the desired confidence level, then the uncertainty in the amplitude measurement Δa_C is given by [Weisskopf et al., 2010], (5.43)

$$\Delta a_C = \sqrt{-\frac{4}{N}ln(1 - C)} \qquad (5.43)$$

The observed amplitude (a) and phase (ψ) on a given confidence contour (C) is expressed in terms of true amplitude (a_o) and phase (ψ_o)o over ϕ which is varied over 0 to 2π is given by [Weisskopf et al., 2010], (5.44) and (5.45)

$$a = (a_o^2 + \Delta a_c^2 + 2a_o\Delta a_c \cos(\phi - \psi_o))^{\frac{1}{2}} \qquad (5.44)$$

$$\psi = \arctan\left(\frac{a - o\sin\psi_o + \Delta a_c \sin\phi}{a_o \cos\psi_o + \Delta a_c \cos\phi}\right) \qquad (5.45)$$

Uncertainty in the measurement increases as the percentage of background counts increases in the measurement. Figure 5.7 shows the relation between the uncertainty and the number of counts for various percentages of background levels. It is observed that high background contributes to high uncertainties in the measurement. As the total number of counts increases the effect of background on the measurement reduces. The uncertainty in a measurement also depends on the true polarization percentage of the source. Figure 5.8 shows the relation between uncertainty and the total number of counts (background neglected) for various cases of true polarization of the source. It is observed that for poor statistics, uncertainty of measurement is high when the true polarization of the source is small. However, as the count-rate increases, uncertainty reduces and becomes independent of true source polarization.

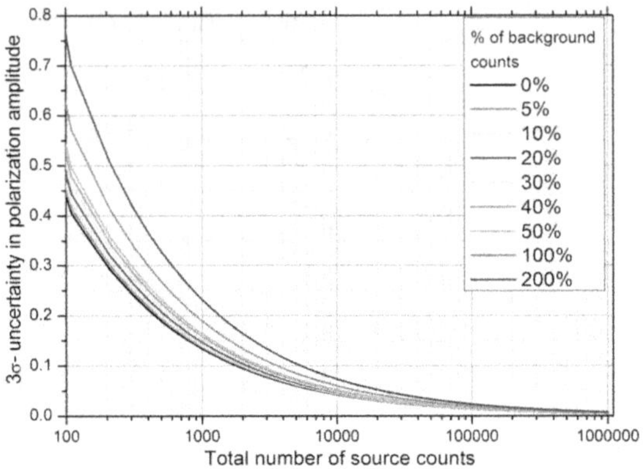

Figure 5.7: $3 - \sigma$ uncertainty in measurement of polarization amplitude as a function of total number of source counts for various cases of background.

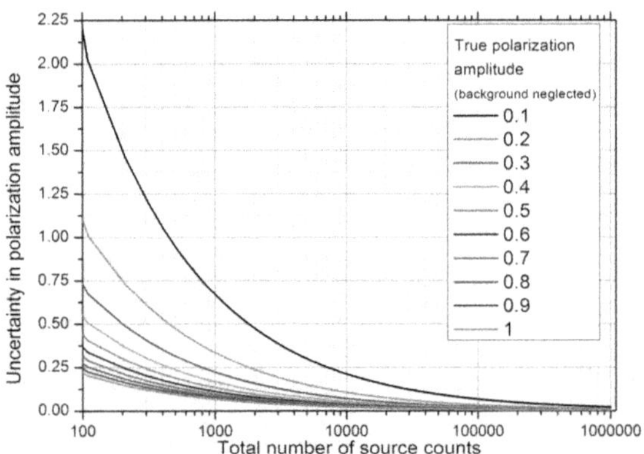

Figure 5.8: $3 - \sigma$ uncertainty in measurement of polarization amplitude as a function of total number of source counts for various cases of true polarization amplitude of the source.

Polarization angle usually follows a normal distribution but the distribution of polarization amplitude is not normal. This is because by the nature, polarization amplitude is always a positive integer. This usually results in the overestimation of amplitude of the polarization percentage for low statistics. This overestimation is also a function of the true degree of polarization i.e. for a given number of source counts, the overestimate of observed polarization is reduces as the true degree of polarization increases. Figure 5.9 shows the relation between the percentage change in the observed polarization as a function of true polarization amplitude. It shows that the overestimate in measurement is high for low true polarization state of the source and for a small number of counts.

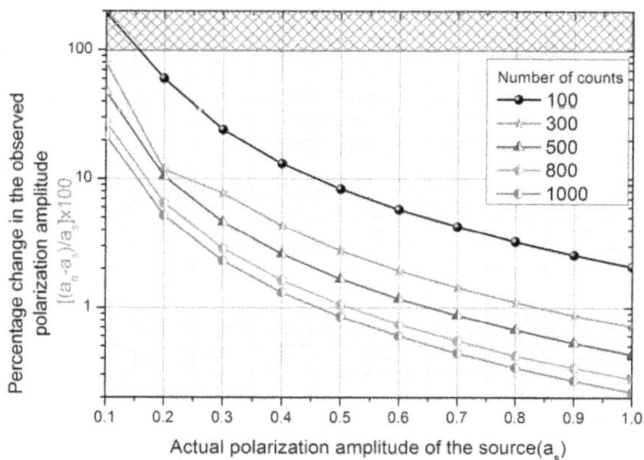

Figure 5.9: Percentage change in the observed polarization amplitude of the measurement as a function of actual polarization amplitude of the source.

5.3.5 Observation in the presence of background

Stokes parameters are additive in nature. Hence the Stokes parameters measured from the source in the presence of background is the sum of Stokes parameters of the source and the background. Hence to avoid the contamination in the measured polarization information of the source, one has to subtract the background

Stokes parameters from the source's Stokes parameters. The background Stokes parameters can be obtained by making an off-source observation of a dark patch of sky close to the target X-ray source. To minimize the statistical errors on the resulting Stokes parameters, we have to subtract the weighted Stokes parameters from the background (weighted with the relative integration time for on-source and off-source) from the source Stokes parameters.

Let t_{off} be the observation time for background and t_{on} is the source observation time, then the background Stokes parameters are weighted with a parameter $w_{off} = -\alpha^{-1}$ where, (5.46) [Kislat et al., 2015]

$$\alpha = \frac{t_{off}}{t_{on}} = \frac{f_{off}}{1 - f_{off}} \tag{5.46}$$

Here f_{off} is the fraction of the total observation time spent off source. Weights on the on- source events will be $w_{on} = 1$. The value of α is decided by the strength of the source and the amount of background present while conducting that particular observation. It is derived as [Kislat et al., 2015], (5.47)

$$\alpha = \frac{R_{BG}}{\sqrt{R_{BG}(R_{BG} + R_S)}} \tag{5.47}$$

where R_{BG} and R_S are expected background and signal rates respectively. If T is the total time of observation then the corresponding MDP(1%) is given by [Kislat et al., 2015], (5.48)

$$MDP = \frac{4.29\sqrt{R_{BG} + R_S}}{\mu\sqrt{T}(R_{BG} + R_S - \sqrt{R_{BG}(R_{BG} + R_S)})} \tag{5.48}$$

5.4 Major science drivers

X-ray polarimetric measurements provide the information on two important parameters of an electromagnetic wave, i.e. polarization amplitude and polarization angle. These parameters provide deep and unique insight to study the behavior of radiation and matter in various physical conditions like extreme magnetic and gravitational fields. X-ray polarimetry also provides a unique platform to test the fundamental physics like observing light bending in the strong gravitational field of a black hole, detect the third order Quantum ElectroDynamic (QED) effects in the magnetosphere of a magnetar, to perform sensitive Lorentz invariance etc. A few important science cases are for X ray polarimetry are discussed below.

Accreting black holes   Thermal emission from the accretion disk around the black hole can be polarized due to Thompson scattering in the disk atmosphere. In the Newtonian plane, the polarization must be either parallel or perpendicular to the disk axis. But due to general relativity effects like the relativistic beaming, frame dragging, etc. the polarization state is altered with respect to that expected from a pure Newtonian case [Dovciak et al., 2008]. Due to general relativity, the radiation undergoes depolarization with respect to an observer at infinity. Effect of returning radiation (radiation emitted from one part of the accretion disk bends and get scattered at other places due to strong gravity) also contributes to the depolarization of the radiation. The effect of depolarization is high in the region close to the black hole. As the temperature of the accretion disk increases with the decrease in the radius, the region close to the black hole usually gets extremely hot and emits X-rays. Hence the depolarization effect is more prominent in X-rays. In Newtonian geometry, the polarization is expected to be constant over the entire energy range. Depolarization of radiation is also a function of the inclination and spin of the black hole. At energies less than 0.1 keV, the degree polarization is same as that of a flat space. But with the increase in energy from 0.1 - 10 keV, polarization decreases. At energies greater than 10 keV, the radiation is from a small area very close to the black hole corona. Since the area of this region is small, the span of change of polarization angle is also small. Hence depolarization effect will be less. At energies greater than 100 keV, the radiation is expected primarily from jets. There also suggestions that this radiation is from the corona of the black hole due to synchrotron emission. Hence the polarization increases at this energies. Hence broad-band X-ray polarization measurements of binary black hole systems can not only constrain the parameters of black hole's inclination, spin, luminosity and emission profile, but also provides an observational evidence to general relativity. Figure 5.10 and figure 5.11 [Schnittman and Krolik, 2009], [Schnittman and Krolik, 2010] shows the simulations of energy dependent polarization degree and angle for two different radiation emission profile, i.e. Noviok-Throne radial emission (a) and power-law emission (a). Figure 5.10 compares the profile for different spins (a/M ratios), where a is the Kerr parameter and M is the mass of the black hole. Figure 5.11 compares the profile for various luminosities (L/L_{Edd}), where L is the luminosity of the source and L_{Edd} is the Eddington luminosity. These simulations suggest that the energy-dependent polarization variation at X-rays have a distinct profile for various black hole parameters and emission mechanisms.

Neutron stars, Magnetors and Pulsars   Compact objects like neutron stars, pulsars and magnetars are expected to be polarized due to the strong magnetic field. The X-ray emission in these type of objects is either due to synchrotron or curvature radiation. The spectra of both synchrotron and curvature radiation are similar whether it is coming from thermal or non-thermal particles particles.Hence

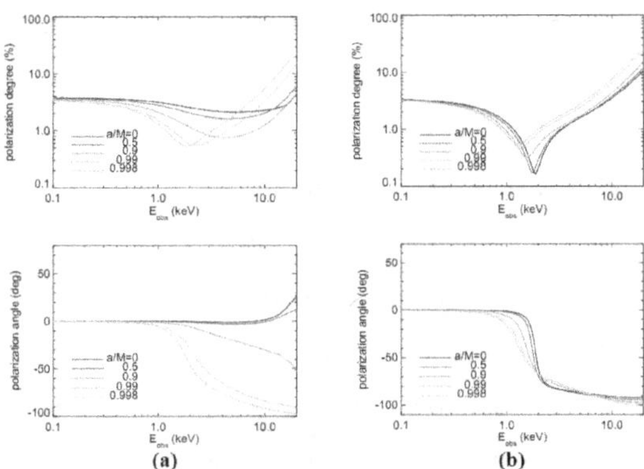

Figure 5.10: Polarization degree and angle for a range of black hole spin parameters. All systems have inclination i = 75°, black hole mass 10$M_\odot$, luminosity L/L_{Edd} = 0.1, for (a) Novikov-Thorne radial emission profiles and (b) Power law emission profile. Reference: [Schnittman and Krolik, 2009]

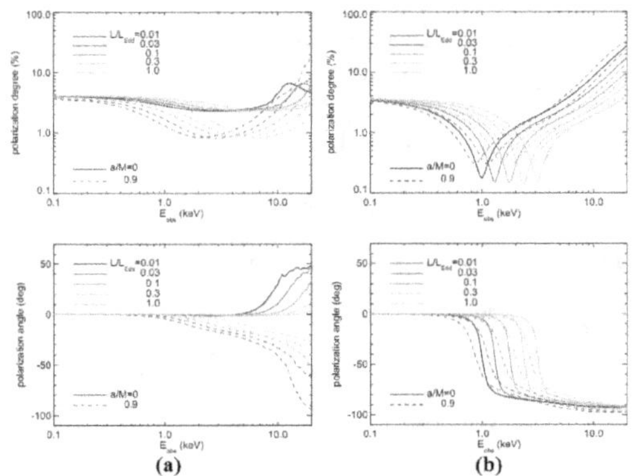

Figure 5.11: Polarization degree and angle for a range of luminosities for a/M = 0 (solid curves)and a/M = 0.9 (dashed curves). All systems have inclination i = 75°, black hole mass 10$M_\odot$, and (a) Novikov-Thorne radial emission profiles (b) Power law emission profile. Reference: [Schnittman and Krolik, 2010]

is it very difficult to distinguish between these two emission mechanisms of a source from only the light-curve and spectroscopic observations. X-ray polarimetric studies can differentiate between these two mechanisms. The degree of polarization of radiation emitted by both mechanisms is also same (usually high). However, the Stokes vectors for synchrotron emission is usually perpendicular to that of curvature radiation. Hence during pulse period, the polarization angle will swing. Curvature pulse polarization angle will show different phase morphology from that of the synchrotron process. Hence in conjunction with light curve and spectroscopy, polarization measurement during pulse period will probe the electron distribution shape and hence suggests the dominant physical process in the object.

X-ray polarization can also a unique technique to distinguish the beam profile of highly magnetic neutron stars (magnetars) [Romani, 1996], [Romani and Watters, 2010]. Figure 5.12 [Schonherr, G. and Wilms, J. and Kretschmar, P. and Kreykenbohm, I. and Santangelo, A. and Rothschild, R. E. and Coburn, W. and Staubert, R.,] shows the schematic of fan beam and pencil beam profile that can exist in a neutron star. In pencil beam profile, the oscillation in the polarization percentage is expected to be out of phase with the pulse, i.e. maximum polarization is expected at the pulse minimum. Whereas in fan beam profile, the percentage of polarization is to be in-phase with the pulse, i.e. maximum polarization at pulse minimum. Hence precise polarization measurement of these objects helps to probe the beam shapes of pulsars. These observations are best suitable around cyclotron resonance frequencies [Schonherr, G. and Wilms, J. and Kretschmar, P. and Kreykenbohm, I. and Santangelo, A. and Rothschild, R. E. and Coburn, W. and Staubert, R.,] usually at 10- 50 keV range).

Active Galactic Nuclei (AGN) AGN emits thermally in the hard-UV band with a peak of thermal emission in the range 30-100 eV with a power law profile extending to X-ray region [Nandra et al., 1991], [Mushotzky et al., 1993]. At

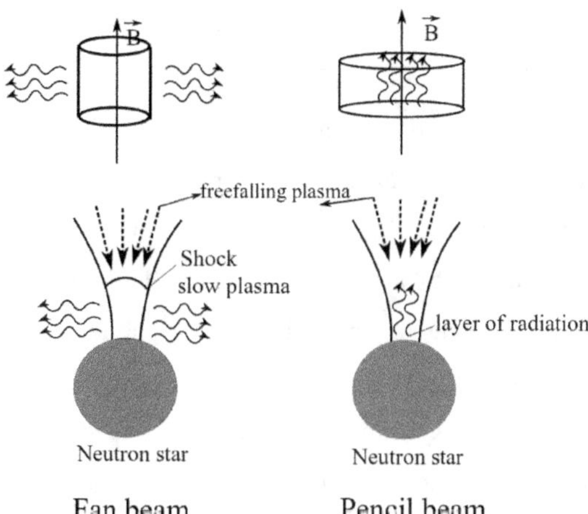

Figure 5.12: Accretion geometries and radiation patterns. Left: "fan beam" (cylinder geometry). Right: "pencil beam" (slab geometry).

hard X-ray region ($100keV$) the coronal emission arises due to comptonization of thermal photons by electrons. This coronal emission is expected to be polarized (8%) [Sunyaev and Titarchuk, 1985], [Schnittman and Krolik, 2010]. Measurement of X-ray polarization at these energies can constrain the inclination of the AGN and also suggests the coronal model of the AGN.

Jets from AGN   Jets in AGN exhibit continuum emission from radio to TeV range. Its spectrum often exhibit a low energy (synchrotron) and a high energy (inverse Compton) peak. Accreting supermassive black holes in AGN with the jet aligned close to the line of sight of observation are called Blazers. The relativistic motion of emission plasma amplifies the jet emission along of line of sight direction and makes blazers very bright. Hence Blazer observation can provide a deep insight into the jet mechanism of an AGN [Krawczynski et al., 2011]. Multi-wavelength polarimetric observations of these objects can provide information regarding how hard X-rays are emitted. There are two different models predicting the emission mechanism at hard X-rays, i.e. Synchrotron Self Compton (SSC) and External Compton models. In SSC model, X-rays come from inverse Compton interactions of electrons with co-spatially emitted synchrotron photons (low energy radiation). In this scenario, one expects the X-ray polarization to be similar to the polarization of low energy radiation (radio, infrared and visible). The degree of polarization this case is usually high. Whereas in external Compton model, the X-ray polarization is expected to be very small ($< 5\%$) [Krawczynski et al., 2011]. Hence X-ray polarimetric measurements in conjunction with polarimetric measurements at other wavelengths can constrain the emission mechanism of hard X-rays in Blazers.

X-ray polarimetry is also an important technique in solar physics to constrain the electron beaming and orientation of the magnetic field with respect to the line of sight. Besides providing a better window in explaining exciting astrophysical problems, X-ray polarimetric studies are also useful in providing a unique platform in testing a few fundamental physical phenomena like testing QED effects in the presence of vacuum birefringence [Baring, 2008], detecting Axion and Axion like particles form highly magnetic sources etc.

5.5 Soft X-ray polarimeter designs

Soft X-ray polarimeter designate operating below 1 keV is uniquely possible by using multilayer mirrors where other techniques are less effective. Recalling equation (2.41) reflected intensity of a multilayer mirrors is given by the equation (5.49).

$$I(\theta) = I_o \mid P^2 + (P^2 - 1)cot^2(A)(P^2 - 1)^{0.5} \mid^{-1} \tag{5.49}$$

where

$A = \frac{2LKd}{m}|F(\theta_m)|,$

$$P = (\tfrac{\pi m L}{2A})[(\theta - \theta_m)sin(2\theta_m) - 2\delta],$$

K $=1$ for $\perp$; $= |cos2\theta_m| for$ $\|$; $= (1+|cos2\theta_m|)/2 for unpolarized light respectively,$

L is the number of layer pairs,

m is the order of Bragg peak,

θ and θ_m are the angle of incidence and the Bragg angle respectively,

$F(\theta_m)$ is the structure function of the coating layer at Bragg angle,

I_o is intensity of incident ray,

δ is real part o refractive index of the material,

d is period of bi-layer of multilayer mirror.

From equation (5.49), one can observe that at $\theta_m = 45^o$ for parallel polarized light, the term 'K' becomes zero which makes the reflected intensity I term zero. In this configuration, the modulation factor of the mirror will be a unity which makes it a perfect polarization analysing element. Figure 5.13 shows the typical reflectivity profile of a multilayer mirror at 45° for S- and P-polarized X-rays. The profile presented in figure 5.13 is a simulated response of a Co-C multilayer mirror with period 3 nm. It is observed that the reflectivity of the multilayer at 45° is negligible for P-polarized X-rays when compared to that of S-polarized X-rays. This difference in the reflectivity value for S- and P- polarized sources is very important for polarization measurements. With this motivation, a couple of polarimeter designs are worked out which are suitable for a small satellite astronomy mission.

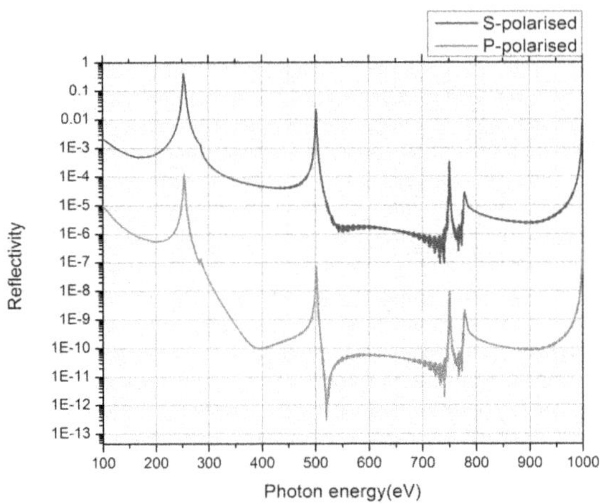

Figure 5.13: Reflectivity profile of a Co-C multilayer at 45° for S- and P- polarized X-rays. These are calculated using IMD software

5.6   Design I: Narrow band soft X-ray polarimeter

The proposed design consists of a single reflection parabolic shell of multilayer mirrors placed at 45° to the incident X-rays. Four pixelated X-ray detectors are placed in the center of the shell such that each detector sees X-rays reflected from each quadrant of the shell. Polarization information is recorded across four detectors simultaneously as a function of azimuthal angle. Figure 5.14 shows the top view and the side view of the mirror and detector structure. Table 5.6 gives the design specifications of the instrument. These parameters are considered in view of a feasible small satellite astronomical polarimetric instrument.

Table 5.1: Specification of the narrowband soft X-ray polarimeter.

Parameter	Specifications
Diameter of the shell	50 cm
Axial profile of the mirror segment	Parabola ($y^2 = 50x$)
Axial length of the mirror	14 cm
Number of detectors	4 (pixelated)
Angle of incidence	45°
Range of incidence angles	40° -50°
Effective geometric area	$1154 cm^2$
Modulation index	0.96
Coating of mirrors	Co-Si
Period of bilayers	2.5 nm
Operation energy	350 eV
Energy spread for non graded coating	330 - 390 eV

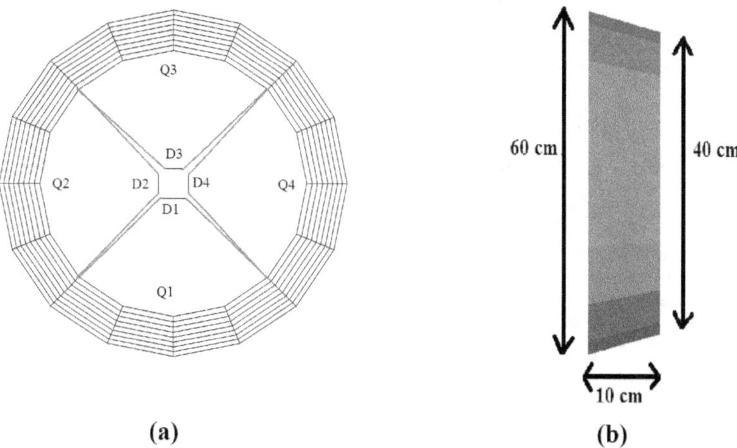

Figure 5.14: (a) Front view of the mirror- detector assembly. (b)Side view of the mirror assembly with dimensions

5.6.1 Mirror profile

Mirror assembly consist of a segmented multilayer mirrors. Number of segments of multilayer mirrors required to complete the mirror assembly depends on the size of the individual segment, which in this case limited with the substrate holder during fabrication in the magnetron sputtering machine. Each mirror segment is a toroidal mirror with circular azimuthal profile and a parabolic axial profile. Parabolic profile reduces the spherical aberration and tightens the spot size. Schematic of an individual mirror segment with dimensions is shown in figure 5.15.

Based on the required sensitivity and optimum possible size of the instrument appropriate for a space instrument, a design with diameter 50 cm is considered with the axial length of each shell as 14 cm. Hence the focal length of the mirror should be 25 cm at the angle of incidence of 45°. The equation of the parabolic profile of mirror which suits above-stated parameters is $Y^2 = 50X$. Figure 5.16 shows the parabolic profile of the mirror with respect to coordinate axis. If the vertex of the parabola is at the origin, then the focus is at the coordinates $(12.5, 0)$ and the mirror is located from coordinates $(8, 20)$ to $(18, 30)$ in parabolic profile. This makes the diameter of the shell as 60 cm at one end of the shell (point 3) and 40 cm at the other end of the shell (point 1).

Arc length of the mirror: Since axial profile of the mirror is a parabola, arc length of the mirror as per figure is the given by the following equation, (5.50)

$$S = \frac{hq}{f} + f \times ln\left(\frac{h+q}{f}\right) \tag{5.50}$$

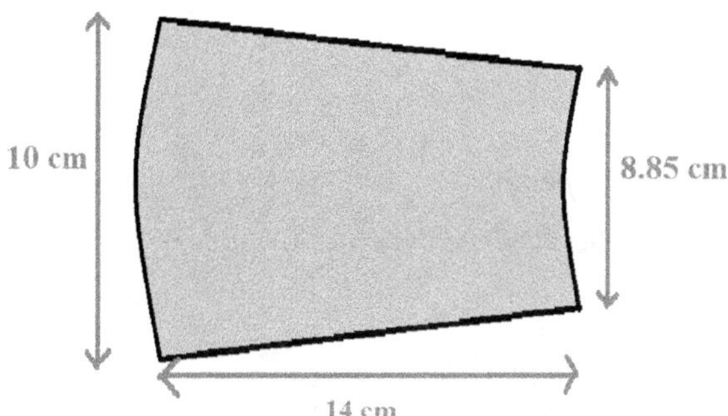

Figure 5.15: Schematic of a single segment of a multilayer mirror with the dimensions

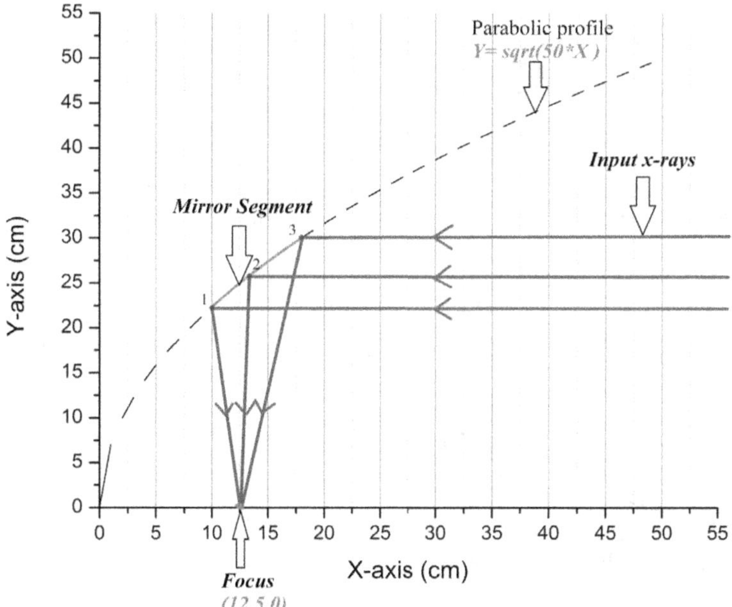

Figure 5.16: Parabolic profile of the mirror.

where

$h = \frac{p}{2}$,

$q = \sqrt{f^2 + h^2}$,

x is any point on the parabola

p is the perpendicular distance from x to the axis symmetry of parabola,

f is the focal length.

Arc length between any two points 1 and 2 on parabola is given by, (5.51)

$$S_1 - S_2 = \frac{h_1 q_1 - h_2 q_2}{f} + f \times ln\left(\frac{h_1 + q_1}{h_2 + q_2}\right) \qquad (5.51)$$

With this equation one can calculate the mirror length if it is parabolic in profile. From the above specified parameters, the arc length of the mirror in this design is 14 cm.

Radius of curvature of the mirror   The radius of curvature of the mirror is not same throughout the axis as the profile is parabolic. There is a gradual and small variation of the radius of curvature of the mirror over the axis of the mirror. Radius of curvature at any point on the curve is given by the standard formula,(5.52)

$$\rho(x) = \frac{(1 + (f'(x))^2)^{\frac{3}{2}}}{f''(x)} \qquad (5.52)$$

where

$\rho(x)$ is the radius of curvature at the point x,

$f(x)$ is the function representing the curve.

For the given equation of a parabola, the radius of curvature of the mirror varies from 95.28 cm at point 3 to 52.50 cm at point 1. Since there is a gradual change in radius of curvature over the mirror, the angle of incidence of input x-rays also slightly deviates from 45°. In this present configuration, the incident angle is around 40° at point 3 and 50° at point 1 as pointed in figure 5.6.1.

5.6.2 Effective area of the Instrument

The geometric area of the mirror assembly is 1550 cm. But the effective area is calculated by multiplying reflectivity of mirrors with the geometric area of the telescope. Peak reflectivity of a typical MCM peaks at a specific energy depends on the coating parameters and the angle of incidence of x-rays onto it. Since there is a gradient change in angle of incidence due to parabolic profile as discussed earlier, reflectivity peak of the overall system also broadened. In the present design due to this broadening, the curve has a flat peak of reflectivity from 330 eV to 390 eV which otherwise should be a sharp peak at 354 eV. Use of laterally graded multilayer mirrors in which the thickness of coating varies across the surface to counter balance the change in angle of incidence can provide a sharp reflectivity peak which improves the energy resolution. Figure 5.6.2 shows the effective area of the instrument with as a function of operational energy.

5.6.3 Performance estimation of the instrument

For an ideal multilayer mirror at 45°, the modulation factor is equal to unity. But in the current configuration, as the angle of incidence of X-rays has a spread (40°-50°) due to curvature, the modulation index of the instrument gets lowered. Figure 6.19 shows the normalized reflectivity of the multilayer as the polarization state of the incident beam varies from P-state (-1) to S-state (+1). When the angle of incidence is exactly equal to 45° the reflectivity at S-state is maximum while it

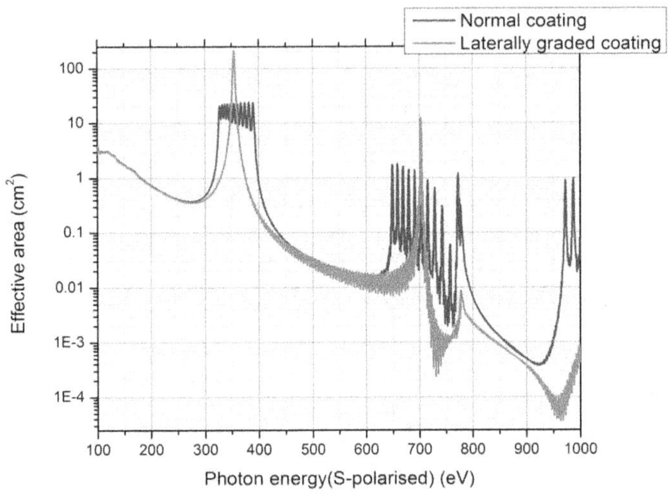

Figure 5.17: Effective area of the system with respect to of incident photon energy. Figure also shows the effective area for two cases when the coating of the mirror is uniform across the surface (blue) and when coated with laterally graded multilayers to counter balance the peak broadening effect from spread in angle of incidence (red).

is zero for P-polarized X-rays, which makes modulation as 1. But in the current configuration, the reflectivity at P-polarized X-rays is slightly greater than zero. Neglecting the background, for the current configuration, the modulation index is expected to be 0.96.

In the current configuration, each detector sees the reflected X-rays over 90° of azimuthal rotation. If the incident X-rays are polarized, an intensity modulation is observed across pixels of each detector. Figure 5.6.3 shows the simulated response of the detector response for the polarized and unpolarized case. It is observed that the intensity inf all detectors remain the same when unpolarized X-rays are incident onto the instrument.

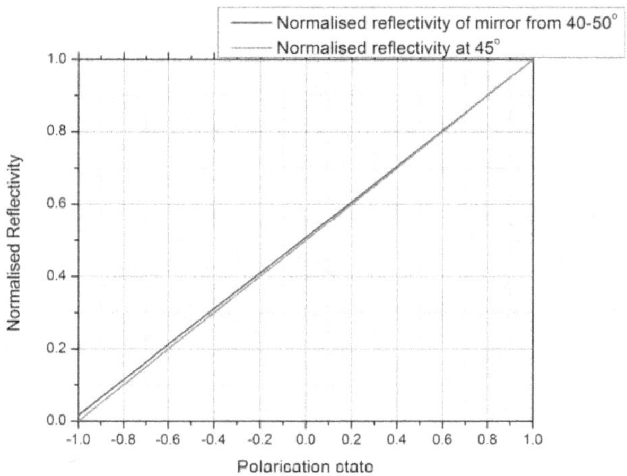

Figure 5.18: Normalized reflectivity of multilayer mirror as a function of polarization state of incident X-rays. In X-axis -1 indicates 100% P-polarized X-rays, +1 indicates 100%S-polarized and 0 indicated unpolarized light

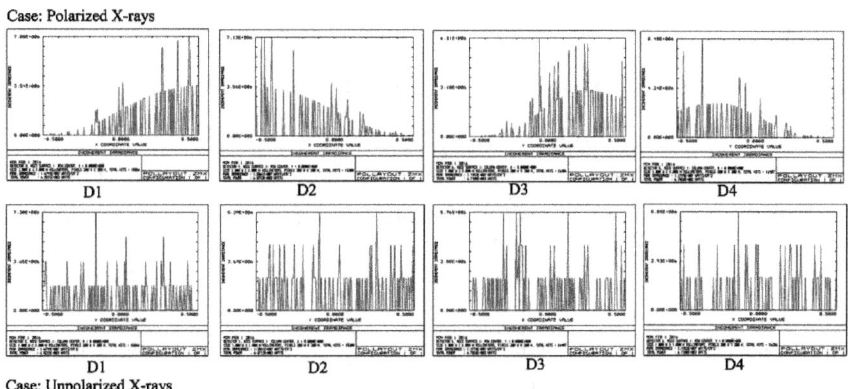

Figure 5.19: Simulated response of instrument's performance for polarized and unpolarized cases.

5.6.4   Discussion

The above-discussed polarimeter operates at 350 eV and has a very high modulation index. The design makes use of four detectors under simultaneous operation which increases the timing property of the instrument. The major disadvantage of this design is its narrowband response which makes it restrictive scientific investigation. Also, use of four detectors simultaneously increases the weight and cost of the instrument. The effective area of the instrument is directly proportional to the diameter of the instrument. Hence as the requirement of the effective area increases, the total volume of the instrument increases proportionally. A requirement of toroidal (parabolic + spherical) segmented multilayer mirrors increases the cost and complexity of the fabrication.

5.7   Design II: Broad band soft X-ray polarimeter

A broad-band soft X-ray polarimeter greatly increases the scientific capacity of the instrument than a narrow band one. Hence an attempt is made to design a broad band instrument using multilayer mirror to operate at energies less than 1 keV [Panini et al., 2018]. The polarimeter consists of three major sub-systems:

- Soft X-ray concentrator.

- Multilayer mirror (one or many on a rotating wheel) placed at 45° with respect to the optical axis of the concentrator.

- A soft X-ray detector positioned at the Nasmyth focus.

The instrument is rotated about its optic axis at a constant rate to derive the intensity modulation for polarized X-rays from the source. If the source is completely unpolarized, the source intensity remains constant during a 180° rotation.

The passband of a fixed period multilayer mirror is usually of the order of a few 10s of eV. In order to increase the overall bandwidth of the instrument, five different multilayer mirrors are arranged at different azimuthal angles, such that only one operates at a time with the detector (fixed). Each mirror's 1st Bragg peak reflectivity is designed to be at different energies spread across the desired energy range. This is analogous to using different filters on an optical telescope. The band-pass of each mirror can be customized by tuning the bi-layer period, the number of bi-layers and the choice of coating materials to get good reflectivity at the 1st Bragg peak. All five mirrors are placed on a motorized rotating platform, that brings each mirror into the converging beam before the focus of the X-ray concentrator, one at a time. For a given multilayer mirror, figure 5.20 shows the schematic of the instrument design with one multilayer mirror in position to reflect X-rays to the detector at the Nasmyth focus. We now present a straw man design for the system and its components.

5.7.1 X-ray concentrator

Use of X-ray concentrator provides the sufficient sensitivity for polarimetric observations. Considering that the instrument should be sensitive to detect the polarization state as low as 2% of at least 200 bright X-ray sources for 100 ks observation, the concentrator would need at least $600 cm^2$ geometric area. Design specification of the concentrator is considered to meet the geometric area requirement and also to have a short focal length ($100 cm$) to make the design compatible with a low-cost space mission. The X-ray concentrator would consist of 24 truncated conical nickel (Ni) coated shells placed in a concentric arrangement. X-rays undergo single grazing angle reflection from the concentrator and converge at the

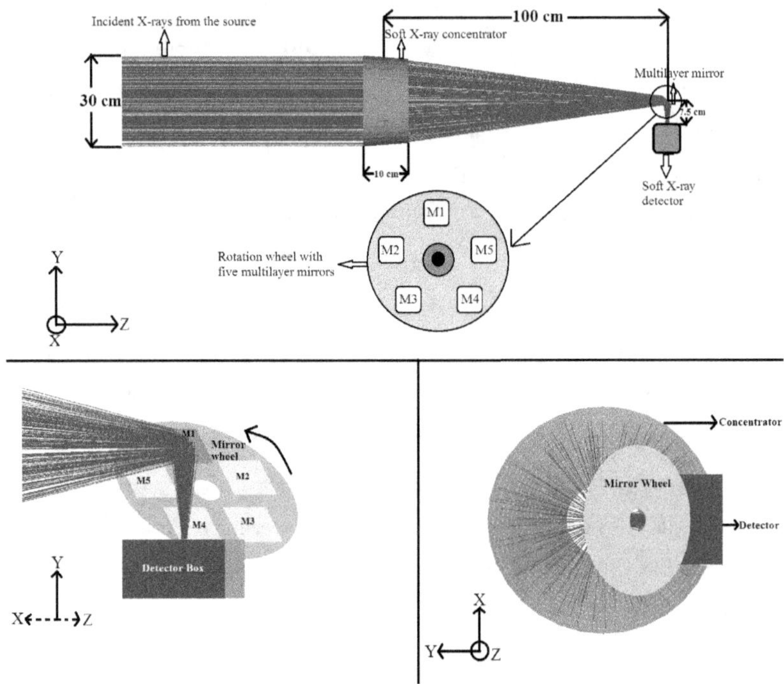

Figure 5.20: **Top**: Optical layout of the soft X-ray polarimeter with a concentrator, polarization analyser (multilayer mirrors) and the detector. **Bottom left**: Zoomed region of the schematic near the focus (axis is rotated by 70° with respect to the coordinates of figure on top. **Bottom right**: Side view of the design (as seen from the prime focus).

focus positioned at a focal length of 107.5 cm. The geometrical area of the concentrator is 630 cm^2. Design specifications of the concentrator are optimized to have high reflection efficiency for X-rays below 1 keV. The radii of the innermost and the outermost shells are 5 cm and 15 cm respectively, and the graze angles of the inner and outermost shells are 1.27^o and 3.84^o respectively. Detailed shell specifications of the concentrator are presented in table 5.7.1. The effective area

(EA) of the concentrator for a given energy 'E' is estimated by summing over the effective areas (geometric area × reflectivity) of all individual shells as given in equation, (5.53)

$$EA_{concentrator}(E) = \sum_{n=1}^{24} 2\pi r_n l \sin(\theta_n) R_n(E, \theta_n) \qquad (5.53)$$

r_n and θ_n are the radii and the axial orientation of the nth shell.'l' is the axial length of the shell. $R_n(E, \theta_n)$ is the reflectivity profile of nth shell as a function of the incident photon energy and θ_n. All reflectivity profiles are calculated using the IMD software within the X-ray oriented programming (XOP) package. Figure 5.21 shows the estimated effective area of the soft X-ray concentrator as a function of the incident photon energy.

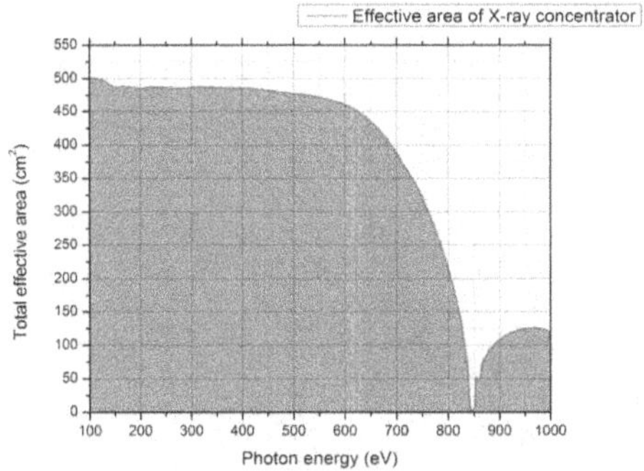

Figure 5.21: Estimated effective area of the concentrator as a function of photon energy. Effective area drops off at 850 eV as the reflectivity of Ni falls rapidly due to the Ni L- shell absorption edge

The substrate of these shells is considered as 0.2 mm aluminium (Al) foils from the heritage of Soft X-ray telescope on board Astrosat. The weight of the optics

Table 5.2: Specifications of the individual shells in the concentrator. r_1 and r_2 are the inner and outer radii of a given shell in the concentrator.

Shell No	Shell No	r_2(cm)	θ (degrees)	Geometrical area (cm^2)	Volume(cm^3)
1	5	4.77	1.27	6.98	6.13
2	5.25	5.02	1.33	7.7	6.44
3	5.51	5.27	1.4	8.5	6.76
4	5.79	5.53	1.47	9.38	7.1
5	6.08	5.81	1.55	10.34	7.46
6	6.39	6.1	1.62	11.4	7.84
7	6.7	6.41	1.7	12.57	8.23
8	7.04	6.72	1.79	13.85	8.64
9	7.39	7.06	1.88	15.25	9.06
10	7.75	7.41	1.97	16.8	9.51
11	8.13	7.77	2.07	18.49	9.98
12	8.53	8.15	2.17	20.36	10.47
13	8.95	8.55	2.28	22.4	10.99
14	9.39	8.97	2.39	24.65	11.52
15	9.85	9.41	2.51	27.11	12.09
16	10.33	9.87	2.63	29.82	12.68
17	10.83	10.35	2.76	32.79	13.29
18	11.35	10.85	2.89	36.06	13.94
19	11.9	11.37	3.03	39.64	14.61
20	12.48	11.92	3.18	43.57	15.32
21	13.08	12.5	3.33	47.88	16.06
22	13.71	13.1	3.5	52.62	16.84
23	14.37	13.7	3.67	57.82	17.65
24	15.06	14.39	3.84	63.52	18.5

without considering support structure is estimated as 733 grams. Aluminium being a low-density metal lowers the weight of the optics which is a major concern for any space-based instrument. At soft X-rays below 0.7 keV optics provides on average effective area of 0.65 $cm^2/grams$. Figure 5.22 shows the effective area contributed by each shell per weight in grams and the total effective area of the concentrator per weight. Table 5.3 summarizes the design specifications of the soft X-ray concentrator.

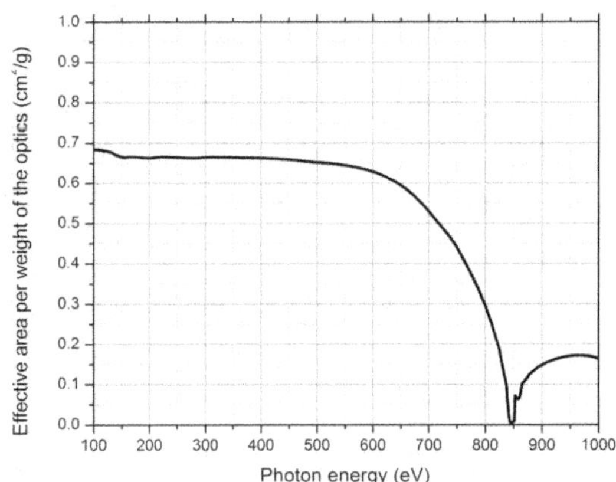

Figure 5.22: Total effective area per total weight of optics of the Soft X-ray concentrator as a function of photon energy.

5.7.2 Multilayer mirrors

All five multilayer mirrors are placed on a motorized wheel such that one multilayer mirror can be operated at a time. The position of multilayer mirror is majorly decided by the maximum size of the footprint of X-rays on the mirror. Experimentally, we have observed that the effective bi-layer period of the multilayer

Table 5.3: Specifications of the soft X-ray concentrator.

Sl.No	Parameter	Quantity
1	Number of shells	24
2	Focal length	110 cm
3	Inner most shell radius	5 cm
4	Outer most shell radius	15.06 cm
5	Axial length of each mirror	10 cm
6	Inner most shell 'θ'	1.27^o
7	Outer most shell 'θ'	3.84^o
8	Coating	Ni
9	Substrate	0.2 mm thick Al foil

mirrors varies laterally over the surface due to fabrication uncertainties. Though this variation is very small (of the order 0.05 nm/cm) for thin multilayers, ideally it is always better to have a small footprint on the multilayer mirror. Figure 5.23 shows the X-ray reflectivity (XRR) test results obtained from a W-B_4C multilayer with 20 bilayers of period 1.7 nm. Red and blue curves represent the XRR test at two different positions on the mirror's surface which are 3 cm away. From these results, the measured effective bi-layer period of red and blue curves are 1.77 and 1.76 respectively. Based on these results, the position of the multilayer mirror is fixed at 100 cm from the X-ray concentrator which corresponds to an elliptical spot of $(2.1 \times 3cm)$ in diameter on the multilayer mirror. From Zemax ray-tracing analysis it is observed that a multilayer mirror of 5 cm in diameter is sufficient to completely receive X-rays from the concentrator even from an off-axis source of $\pm 0.3^o$.Specifications of the multilayer mirrors are given in table 5.4. The ratio of the thickness of the metallic layer (high Z-element) to the total thickness of a bi-layer is set to 0.4 for all coatings.

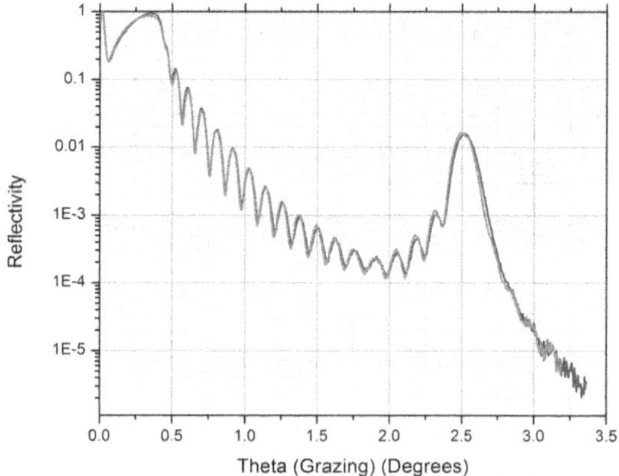

Figure 5.23: X-ray reflectivity measurements at 8.047 keV of a W-B_4C multilayer mirror with 20 bi-layers of period 1.7 nm at two different positions which are 3 cm away. The measured bi-layer period of red and blue curves are 1.77 and 1.76 nm respectively

5.7.3 Soft X-ray photon counting detector

The soft X-ray detector is placed at the Nasmyth focus, 7.5 cm away from the multilayer mirror. The detector is expected to have good quantum efficiency ($\geq 20\%$) at low energy X-rays (< 0.5 keV) which is a challenge as the optical light rejection window absorbs soft X-rays at these wavelengths. High spectral resolution of the detector is not a primary requirement as the multilayer mirrors reflect only a narrow band of energies but may be very useful for background rejection.

5.7.4 Optics performance

Since the front optics consists of single reflection conical shells, the design has a very poor imaging quality and hence suitable only for non-imaging polarimetry. Imaging is severely limited by coma aberration for off-axis sources. Figure 5.24 shows the Zemax ray-tracing simulations of the optical design. It is observed that

Table 5.4: Specifications of multilayer mirrors on the mirror wheel.

Mirror ID	Coating	Period of bi-layers (nm)	Energy of 1st Bragg peak
M1	W-Si	1.5	587
M2	Ni-Si	1.8	490
M3	Ni-Si	2.3	384
M4	Co-C	2.9	306
M5	Co-C	3.5	254

off-axis point sources have a spread in the image plane which resembles the coma aberration. Field of view of the instrument is $\pm 0.3^{o}$ for a 1 cm $\times$ 1 cm detector. Figure 5.25 shows the collimator response (normalized effective area Vs off-axis angle) of the design. Though the off-axis image quality of the system is very poor, the polarization measurement of an off-axis point source will not have additional modulation from aberrations since the collimator response is symmetric about the optical axis.

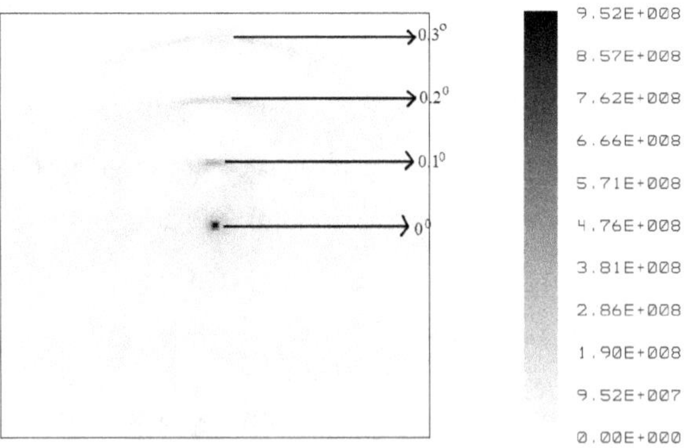

Figure 5.24: Zemax ray-tracing simulations of the optical performance. 4 point sources are placed, one at on-axis and other at off axis positions of 0.1^{o}, 0.2^{o} and 0.3^{o}.

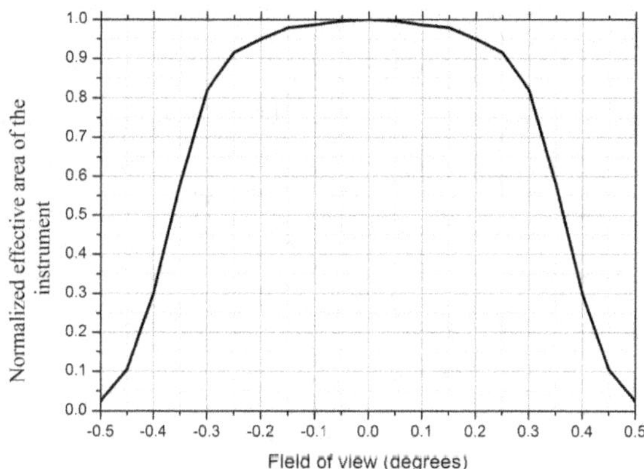

Figure 5.25: Normalized effective area of the instrument as a function of the off-axis angle (collimator response).

5.7.5 Estimated performance analysis of the Instrument

The effective area of the instrument depends on the effective area of the X-ray concentrator, the reflectivities of multilayer mirrors and the efficiency of the detector system. The converging X-rays from the exit pupil of the concentrator are incident on the multilayer mirror at a range of angles. Since the reflectivity of the multilayer mirror and the energy of the Bragg peak depend on the angle of incidence, the overall response of the instrument depends on the $F_{\#}$ (ratio of focal length to the diameter of the outermost shell) of the concentrator. The concentrator consists of 24 shells with a maximum diameter of the exit pupil of 30 cm and focal length of 107.5 cm. As shown in figure 5.20, the concentrator's entrance aperture defines the x-y plane and the +z axis points towards the multilayer mirror. A multilayer mirror is placed at 45° to the optical axis of the concentrator as shown in figure   5.20.The beam of converging X-rays from 37° to 58° depending on y coordinate along the concentrator. X-rays incident at 45° are reflected from the y=0 plane of the concentrator, 37° from the y=-15 plane and 58° are from the y=+15 plane. Equation (5.54) gives the grazing angle (in degrees) on the multilayer as a function of y. The geometric area as a function of Y is shown in figure 5.26(left). Figure 5.26(right) shows the front view of the concentrator seen from the source end marked at different positions along the y-axis.

$$\theta = tan^{-1}\left(\frac{y}{f}\right) + 45^o \tag{5.54}$$

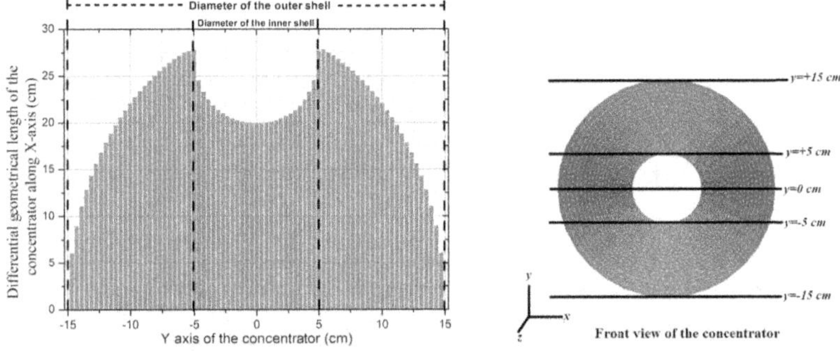

Figure 5.26: **Left**:Geometric length of the concentrator along X-axis as a function of the concentrator position. The central dip is due to the unfilled inner region of the innermost concentrator.**Right** : Front view of the concentrator (seen from the source end) marked at different positions along y-axis.

The geometric length of the concentrator falls to zero at y=$\pm$ 15 (maximum radius of the concentrator). The central dip from $\pm$ 5 cm corresponds to the unfilled inner 10 cm diameter of the concentrator. Overall reflectivity at a given y-plane of the concentrator is calculated as the average reflectivity from all shells contributing to the reflection at that plane. At y=0 all 24 shells contribute to X-ray reflection but at y=±15 only the outer shell contributes. The reflectivity profile of the concentrator varies with y symmetrically about the y=0 plane (figure 5.27 left). Figure 5.27 (right) shows the reflectivity profile as a function of Y-axis of the concentrator at two energies. This profile is symmetric about y=0 plane of the concentrator.

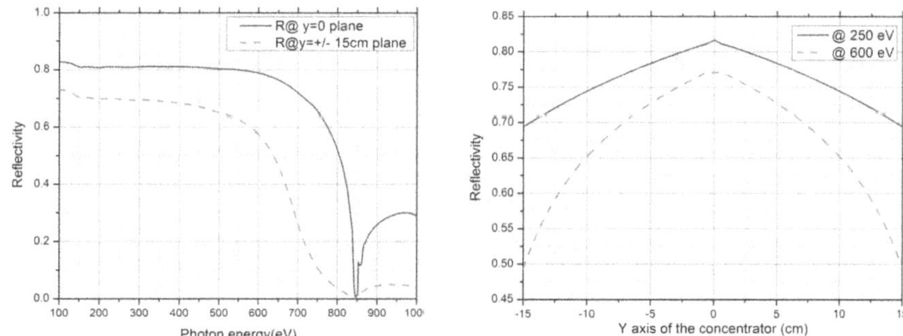

Figure 5.27: **Left**: Comparison of effective reflectivity of the concentrator at y=0 and y=±15 cm. **Right**: Reflectivity of the concentrator as a function of the Y-axis at 250 eV and 600 eV

To estimate the effective area of optics, the reflectivity of the multilayer mirror at an angle is multiplied by the effective area of the concentrator. By design, the angle at which X-rays fall on the multilayer mirror depends on the the value of y along the concentrator and the total effective area of the optics (EA) is, (5.55)

$$EA_{optics} = \int_{y=-15}^{y=+15} R_{\theta(y)}^{ml}(e) \times EA(y)dy \qquad (5.55)$$

Table 5.5:   Bandpass, width, and grasp of the instrument with individual multilayer mirrors in place.

Mirror ID	Band of operation (eV)	Band width (eV)	Grasp ($cm^2 eV$)
M1	520-685	165	200
M2	435-570	135	160
M3	340-450	110	210
M4	270-360	90	340
M5	220-300	80	520

where $R_{\theta(y)}^{ml}(e)$ is the reflectivity of the multilayer mirror at a given angle which corresponds to the y-plane of the concentrator as given in equation (5.53). EA(y) is the effective area of the concentrator which is a product of differential geometric area and reflectivity of the concentrator at a given y (as shown in figure 5.26(left)). The reflectivities of all multilayer mirrors are calculated assuming the RMS surface roughness to be 0.5 nm and an interlayer roughness of 0.1 nm per layer. Since the reflectivity is integrated over the y-axis, the spread in incidence angles of X-rays leads to broadening of the Bragg peak, but integrated sensitivity remains unchanged for continuum sources.

Figure 5.28 shows the effective area of the optics as a function of photon energy for all five multilayer mirrors which are to be operated individually, one at a time. Table 5.6 summarizes the operational band of each mirror and the total "grasp" (grasp= effective area × bandwidth).

Figure 5.29 shows the effective area of the instrument for S- and P-polarized X-rays. The grasp of the instrument is around 50 times more for S-polarized X-rays than for P-polarized.

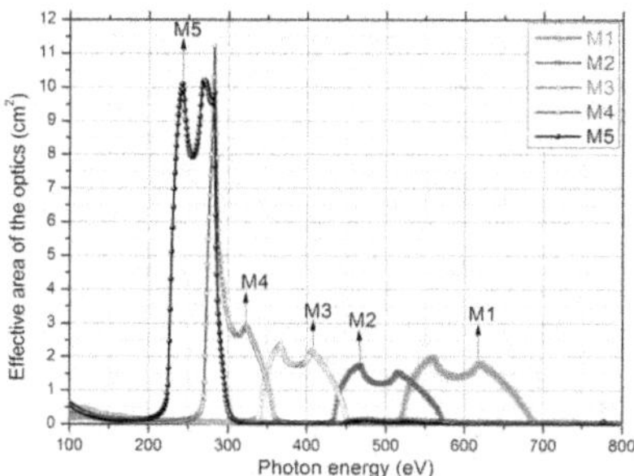

Figure 5.28: Effective area of optics for unpolarized X-rays as a function of photon energy for all five mirrors.

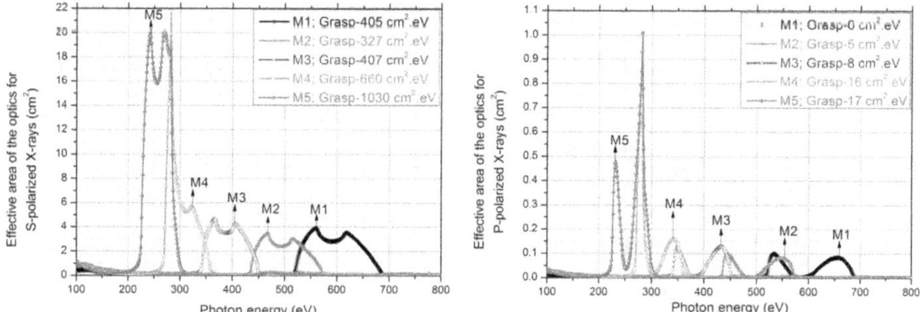

Figure 5.29: **Left**: Maximum effective area of the optics (achieved for 100 % polarized X-rays in s-polarized state). **Right**: Minimum effective area of the optics (achieved for 100 % polarized X-rays in p-polarized state)

5.7.6 Modulation factor

The intensity of a linearly polarized X-ray source modulates at double the frequency of azimuthal rotation of the instrument. The modulation factor (μ) is an important parameter of a polarimeter which is defined by equation (5.56). $\mu = 1$ for an ideal polarimeter. A multilayer mirror at 45° acts as a perfect X-ray polariser. But in this design, rays are incident on the multilayer mirror over a range of angles around 45°. From figure 5.29(right) it is observed that the effective area of the mirror for p-polarized light goes to zero only at the central wavelength (corresponds to reflectivity at 45°) of a band and gradually increases away from this central wavelength.

$$\mu = \frac{S_{max} - S_{min}}{S_{max} + S_{min}} \tag{5.56}$$

S_{max} and S_{min} are the maximum and minimum intensities of a completely polarized source seen through the polarimeter, separated by 90° of azimuthal rotation. Figure 5.30 shows the modulation factor of the instrument as a function of incident photon energy for all mirrors. The modulation factor of the instrument is over 0.9 for all bands. Since the flux is integrated over the pass-band of the spectrum (see table 5.6) and the shape of modulation factor varies over that range, the overall modulation of the instrument is calculated using the grasp for each mirror. Table 5.6 summarizes the modulation factor of the instrument in each band. If G_S and G_P are grasps of the instrument for a particular multilayer mirror at its 1st Bragg peak, then the modulation factor is given by equation (5.57). This equation assumes that the spectrum of the source and the quantum efficiency of the detector are uniform over the spectral band.

$$\mu = \frac{G_S - G_P}{G_S + G_P} \tag{5.57}$$

5.7.7 Instrumental polarization from the soft X-ray concentrator

Instrumental polarization is defined as the intrinsic modulation induced within the instrument for unpolarized incident light. In this design, instrumental polarization

Table 5.6: Operational band and grasp of the instrument for s- and p- polarized X-rays with respect to the multilayer mirror and the effective modulation factor of the instrument for a band.

Mirror ID	Band of operation (eV)	G_S $(cm^2 eV)$	G_p $(cm^2 eV)$	μ
M1	520-685	405	6	0.97
M2	435-570	327	5	0.97
M3	340-450	407	8	0.96
M4	270-360	660	16	0.95
M5	220-300	1030	17	0.96

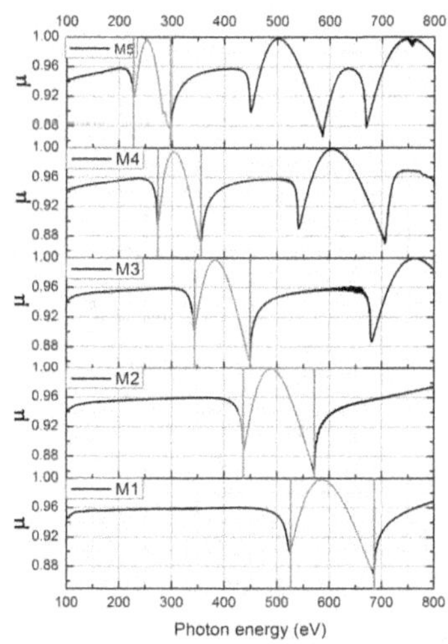

Figure 5.30: Modulation factor of the polarimeter optics as a function of incident photon energy for all five mirrors. Selected regions in red represent the bands of operation in which the mirror is designed to be operated.

can mainly occur due to the difference in S- and P-polarized X-ray reflectivities from the soft X-ray concentrator. Currently used soft X-ray detectors are polarization insensitive. Instrumental polarization can adversely affect the measured degree of polarization and polarization angle. For a closed shell X-ray concentrator which integrates X-rays reflected from all azimuthal angles equally, the net change in polarization angle due to instrumental effects is zero. This can be understood if we examine the Muller matrix of the X-ray concentrator as a function of incident photon energy. The Muller matrix for such a setup reduces to a diagonal matrix after 360° azimuthal integration of flux and is given by [Almeida and Pillet, 1993], (5.58)

$$M = 0.5(1 - \epsilon^2) \times \begin{bmatrix} A + B & 0 & 0 & 0 \\ 0 & A & 0 & 0 \\ 0 & 0 & A & 0 \\ 0 & 0 & 0 & A - B \end{bmatrix} \tag{5.58}$$

where $A = |R_s + R_p|^2$, $B = |R_s - R_p|^2$ and R_s and R_p are the reflectivities of the mirror for s- and p- polarized X-rays respectively. ϵ is the centre obscuration ratio between the internal and external radii of the annular aperture. It is a measure of the active area from where rays are reflected. As the Muller matrix is only a diagonal matrix, there is no cross-talk between the two polarization states of incident X-rays. If the reflection efficiency of the concentrator is same for both S- and P- polarized X-rays, then the Muller matrix becomes an identity matrix which acts as an attenuator. The residual instrumental polarization of the concentrator is given by [Almeida and Pillet, 1993], (5.59)

$$IP = \frac{(R_s - R_p)^2}{(R_s + R_p)^2} \tag{5.59}$$

The instrumental polarization of the soft X-ray concentrator is calculated by determining the S- and P- polarized reflectivities from an individual shell as a function of incident photon energies and then computing the same for the complete system. Figure 5.31 shows the residual instrumental polarization calculated as per equation (5.59) as a function of photon energy for the soft X-ray concentrator. As the instrumental polarization of the concentrator is very low (of the order of 10^{-5}), it can be neglected for practical purposes as the sensitivity of the polarization analysing mirrors is much larger.

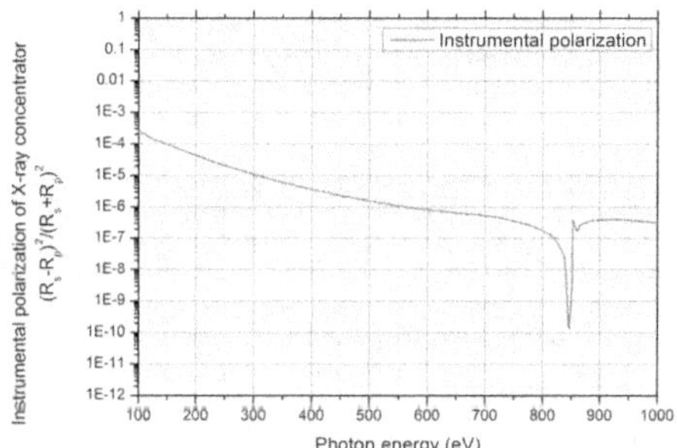

Figure 5.31: Residual instrumental polarization of the soft X-ray concentrator as a function of incident photon energy.

Instrumental polarization may occur when there is a mismatch in the optical axis of the concentrator and the axis of rotation of the instrument. Maximum efforts need be made to ensure required alignment is reached during ground integration. However, various scenarios (including pre-launch vibration, launch, separation shock, etc) could create misalignment. For an on-axis point source, with no instrumental misalignment, the angle of incidence of the chief ray from the concentrator to the multilayer mirror is 45° and is constant over the rotation of the instrument. But if the axis of the rotation has a constant misalignment of angle θ with respect to the optical axis, the chief ray from the concentrator makes an angle $45^o \pm \theta$ with the multilayer mirror. This will result in a change in the modulation factor of the instrument. However, this can be eliminated largely using on-board calibration with a known unpolarized cosmic source and correcting the final results for the intrinsic modulation arising from of the instrument.

5.7.8 Instrument sensitivity

The concentrator allows the instrument to gather more flux from a source relative to background and hence improves the MDP of the instrument. The MDP of the instrument was estimated for several bright sources by considering their soft X-ray flux from the XMM-Newton catalog [Rosen. et al., 2016]. There are at least 100 sources which are bright enough whose MDP is less than 2% at 99% confidence for 100 ks of integration time per band. For this calculation, we assume that the detector has a quantum efficiency of 70% in the whole band. Background counts are mainly contributed by the cosmic soft X-ray background and detector background. Soft X-ray background from extragalactic sources from 0.1-2 keV follows a power law with index $\tau=1.46\pm0.06$ and normalization factor A=10.5 keV $cm^{-2}\ s^{-1}\ sr^{-1}\ keV^{-1}$. This is approximately 65 counts per 100 ks observation time which is 10% of the source counts expected in the given operation band of the instrument for most bright sources of interest. Internal background counts from the detector are mainly due to the readout noise and the thermal noise of the detector. Detector noise can be lowered by cooling the system and is usually very low when compared to the cosmic soft X-ray background. The MDP of the instrument is different at different energies as the effective area of the instrument, and the source flux varies as a function of the photon energy. Table 5.7 gives, estimated MDP values for the blazar PKS 2155-304 for a 100 ks integration time. For these estimations, we have considered 10% (i.e. b=0.1×r) of total counts received arises from background sources.

Table 5.7: Estimated MDP of values for the blazar PKS 2155-304 in 100 ks integration per band with 10% background counts using different multilayer mirrors.

Mirror ID	M1	M2	M3	M4	M5
Energy band (eV)	520-685	435-570	340-450	270-360	220-300
MDP (%) at 99% confidence for 100 ks	0.62	0.60	0.40	0.29 9	0.17

5.7.9 Discussion

The soft X-ray polarimeter design proposed in this paper has a broadband sensitivity to soft X-rays less than 1 keV. The estimated modulation factor at each band is over 0.9 which provides good polarization detection sensitivity. Multilayer mirrors used in this design are small in dimensions (3×3 cm), have a uniform period coating, and plane mirrors. Hence it is relatively easy to fabricate such mirrors. As the design requires a single detector to detect the polarization state of input X-rays, the power and weight requirement of the system is minimized. However, the instrument must be rotated continuously to provide the signal modulation. And also the multi-band polarization measurements require switching between multilayer mirrors faster than the source variability time scale. Instrument polarization from the concentrator is estimated to be under 10^{-5} over the operational band. Hence the design is ideally suited for sensitive polarimetric studies of cosmic X-ray sources. The sensitivity of the instrument can be scaled up or scaled down just by changing the number of shells in the concentrator without any significant change in the dimensions of the instrument.

5.8   Simultaneous broad-band soft X-ray polarimeter

One of the major disadvantages of the polarimeter in design II is that the broad-band observations is not simultaneous. While each multilayer mirror completely uses the total effective area of the concentrator, the instrument has to operate in 5 different bands in-order to cover the entire spectrum. The design also requires a rotating wheel which increases the complexity for a space instrument. With some minor modifications in the design, the instrument can operate simultaneously in the entire spectrum. This can be achieved by developing a mosaic multilayers with different periods. A mosaic multilayer mirror can be prepared by carefully cutting different multilayer mirrors and arranging them into a single mosaic mirror. Figure 5.32 shows schematic of the polarimeter with a mosaic multilayer mirror for simultaneous broad band observation. In this design, the total effective area of the concentrator is divided by each multilayer mirror to reflect soft X-rays of different energies.

The major advantage of this modification to a soft X-ray polarimeter is the simultaneous observation of the source from 0.2 keV to 0.7 keV. Since a single mosaic multilayer mirror is used as a polarizing element, no mechanism for a rotating mirror wheel is required. This reduce the weight and complexity of the entire system. However, in this configuration each energy band operates a small portion of the concentrator's effective area, the overall observation time per energy increases. This limits the observation of highly variable X-ray sources whose flux variability is of the order of observation time required for polarization measurement.

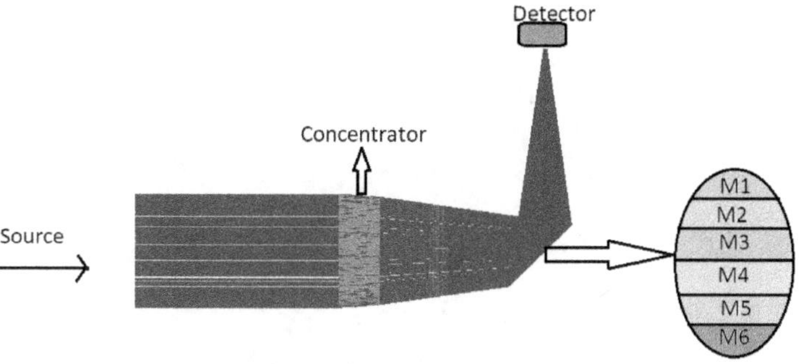

Figure 5.32: Schematic of the simultaneous broad-band polarimeter design with a single mosaic multilayer mirror as a polarizing element.

5.9 Summary

In this chapter we have summarized the important science motivations for soft X-ray polarimetry and also presented a quick review on the available techniques and limitations for astronomical X-ray polarimetry. We have presented two design concepts soft X-ray polarimeters based on multilayer mirrors. We have also estimated the performance of these designs. These instruments works as polarimeters less than 1 keV. Multilayer mirror based polarimeters have very high modulation factor (> 0.9) hence they are very efficient. We have also proposed alternative design for simultaneous broadband observation of soft X-ray polarization.

Chapter 6

Development of thin substrate multilayer mirrors through ion etching

6.1   Motivation

The soft X-ray broad-band polarimeter described in Chapter 5 can also be implemented as an additional back-end instrument for a hard X-ray telescope. A conceptual design of a broadband hard X-ray polarimeter is under study phase for future Indian astronomical instrument. A proposal was made by combining the multilayer mirror based soft X-ray polarimeter and Compton scattering based hard X-ray polarimeter as back-end instruments with a hard X-ray telescope at the front-end. Schematic of this instrument is given in figure 6.1.

The instrument consists of a depth-graded multilayer mirror based hard X-ray telescope at the front-end and two simultaneous back end instruments for soft and hard X-ray polarimetry. Depth-graded multilayer mirror based hard X-ray telescope focuses X-rays from very small energies (< 1 keV) to hard X-ray

$\sim$ 100 keV. Soft X-ray polarimeter works less than 1 keV similar to the design discussed in chapter 5. Compton scattering polarimeter acts as a polarimeter at hard X-rays above 15 keV. Soft X-rays from the telescope reflects from the multilayer mirror and focuses on to the soft X-ray detector at the Nasmyth focus. Hard X-rays gets transmitted through the multilayer mirrors and gets focussed onto the Compton scattering element at the prime focus. This setup provides simultaneous observations to both soft and hard X-rays. The major advantage of this design is that the total effective area of the telescope is used by both instruments simultaneously as they operate as different energy ranges.

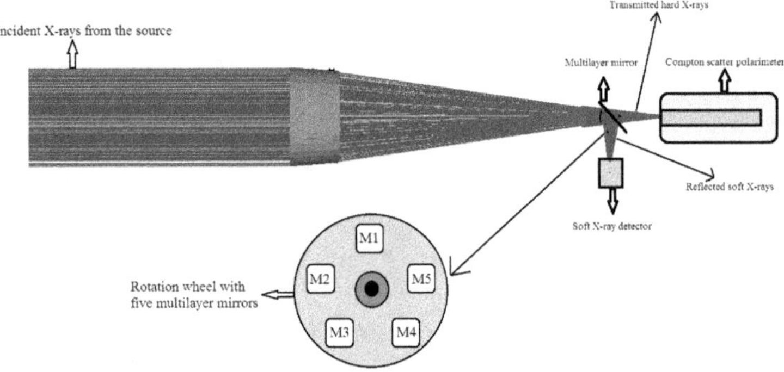

Figure 6.1: Schematic of a broad-band X-ray polarimeter with a combination of a multilayer mirror based soft X-ray polarimeter and a Compton scattering based hard X-ray polarimeter as the back-end instruments with a depth-graded multilayer mirror based hard X-ray telescope at the front end.

6.1.1 X-ray absorption from the substrate

The major challenge in implementing this instrument is the absorption of X-rays by the substrate of multilayer mirrors. The standard substrate we use for depositing multilayer structure is 500 microns thick super polished Silicon (Si). While hard X-rays above 15 keV can get transmitted with high efficiency ($>65\%$) from the multilayer film (~ 0.2 microns), they significantly get absorbed at the thick Si substrate. This reduces the effective area of the instrument for hard X-ray polarimeter at energies from 15 keV to 25 keV. X-ray absorption can be reduced by using ultra-thin substrates (~ 100 microns). However, handling such thin substrates is difficult. Figure 6.2 shows the transmission efficiencies of W/B_4C multilayer mirrors with period 2 nm and 100 number of bi-layers at 45° degrees with different substrate thickness as a function of photon energy. It is observed that the transmission efficiency is only 20% at 15 keV for 500 microns thick substrate while it is 70 % for 100-micron thick substrate.

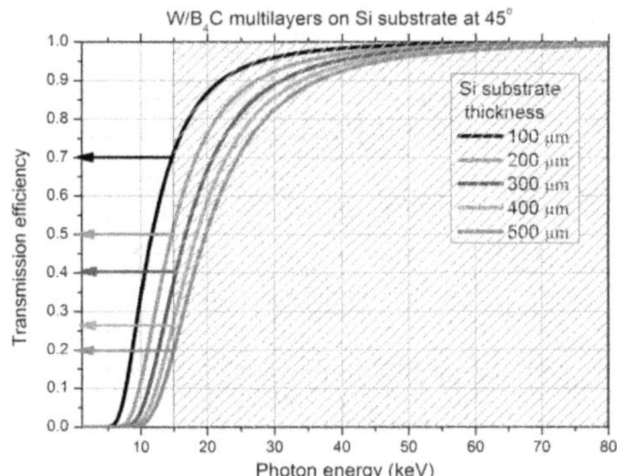

Figure 6.2: The transmission efficiencies of W/B_4C multilayer mirrors with period 2 nm and 100 number of bi-layers at 45° degrees with different substrate thickness as a function of photon energy.

The major challenge in developing thin substrate multilayer mirrors lies in the mechanical and thermal stability of the mirror. In order to reduce substrate thickness from finished multilayer mirrors coated on thicker Si, initiated a process for localized Silicon etching of the substrate. By this technique, we etched approximately 400 microns of Si from the substrate from the non-reflective surface of the mirror. Silicon etching can also be done only at a specific portion of the substrate where hard X-rays are expected to be transmitted. This does not significantly alter the mechanical stability of the mirror as the major portion of the mirror is left with a thick substrate. We conducted Si etching of our samples at the Laboratory for Electro-Optical System (LEOS), Indian Space Research Organisation (ISRO), Bengaluru.

6.2 Silicon etching through Deep Reactive Ion Etching

Etching is a chemical process to remove layers of micron sized thickness from the surface. Etching is a very popular technique in developing Micro-Electro-Mechanical Systems (MEMS). When a silicon substrate is subjected to a specific liquid chemical or a vapour plasma (etchant), the microlayers on the substrate get etched out. Etching is broadly classified into two types: Wet etch and Dry etch. Wet etch uses liquid chemicals to remove materials from the wafer. In dry etching, material removal is done using energetic plasma. Different etchants are used for removal of different materials. For most applications, only a specific pattern of the substrate needs removal. In order to achieve this a photo-resist mask is coated on the wafer in the desired pattern. Photo-resist material is immune to etchant materials hence etching does not happen at photo-resist layers. The flow chart for the patterned dry etching process is described in the figure 6.3.

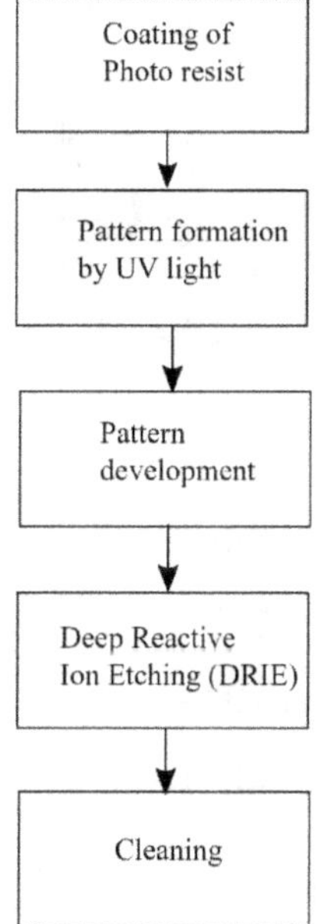

Figure 6.3: Flow chart describing the patterned dry etching process.

We have performed patterned Silicon dry etching technique on the non-reflecting side of multilayer mirrors. We etched 400 microns out of a 500 micron thick substrate in a circular pattern of diameter 5 mm. Figure 6.4 shows the schematic of a the whole Si etching process including photo-resist pattern development, Dry etching and cleaning process.

6.2.1   Coating photo-resist layer

Photo-resist layer is coated on the rear side of the multilayer mirror using spin coating. In order to perform spin coating, the mirror is heated to $\sim 80^{o}$ C and

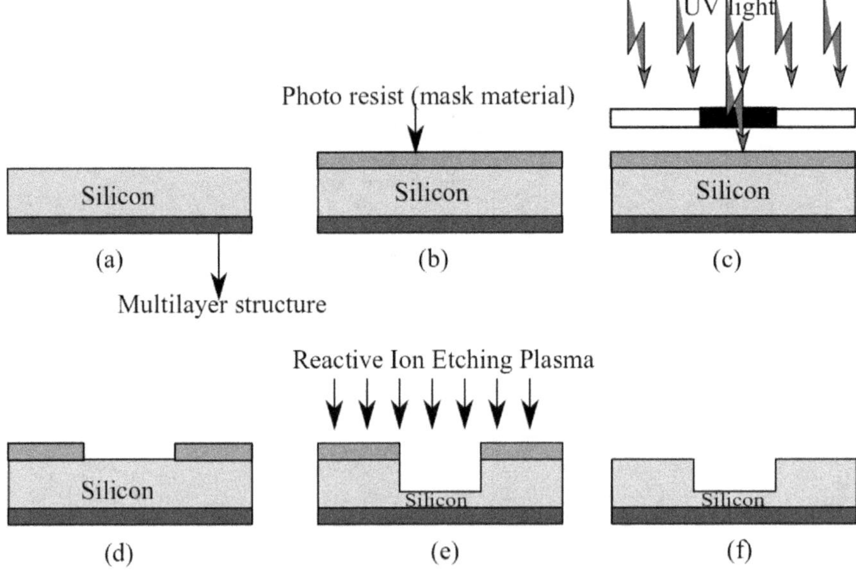

Figure 6.4: Schematic of Si etching process on the rare side of a multilayer mirror.

wax applied on the multilayer film side. The wax acts as epoxy which helps to keep the substrate attached to the rotating platform during spin coating. We used 555-HMP-1116 of $AREMCO^{TM}$ as wax for adhesion. The substrate is attached to glass slate which is placed on a rotating platform for spin coating. We have used Polyamide-AZ10XT $(520CP)^{TM}$ (1 Methonal 2-Proposal acetone (108-65-6)) as a photo-resist layer. A solution of photo-resist is applied on the substrate and the substrate is spun at a speed of 1000 RPM for 30 seconds at room temperature and pressure. This forms a uniform photo-resist layer of 10 microns across the surface. The thickness of the layer is inversely proportional to the square root of the rotation speed. After spin coating, the substrate is heated to 80° C for 40 minutes.

6.2.2   Pattern formation

Photoresist is removed from the substrate in a desired pattern before the start of etching process. A photomask is developed in the required pattern. In this case, the pattern is a circular aperture of diameter 5 mm. The photomask efficiently absorbs the Ultra-Violet (UV) light all across the surface except at the aperture. The photomask is placed on the substrate and the whole setup is exposed to UV light for 135 seconds. UV light breaks the polymer bonds of the photo-resist material in the vicinity of the aperture. After UV exposure, the substrate is cleaned with the developer solution. Cleaning with developer solution removes the photoresist layer whose bonds are broken due to UV exposure.35 mL developer (Hydride de Potassium) ($AZ400k^{TM}$) is mixed with 65 mL of distilled water to make a developed solution. After thoroughly cleaning the substrate with the developer solution, the substrate is baked for 15 minutes at 70° C. This process develops the pattern in the photo-resist layer on the substrate.

6.2.3   Deep Reactive Ion Etching (DRIE)

Deep Reactive Ion Etching (DRIE) is a dry etching process where ion plasma is used to etch the material from the substrate. We have used dry O_2, SF_6 and C_4F_8 plasma for etching process. In order to get the anisotropic etch, we used Bosh process for etching. Anisotropic etch allows the etch process occur only in one axis i.e. in the axis vertical to the substrate. In Bosh process, C_4F_8 plasma acts as a passivation layer and SF_6 plasma acts as etching plasma. For each cycle of etching, C_4F_8 layer is deposited on the substrate alternating with SF_6 plasma. SF_6 plasma etches the pre-existing C_4F_8 layer and then etches some portion of Silicon. Residual C_4F_8 layer restricts the Si etching across the walls allowing only etching only in one direction. This process is repeated several times until Si etching process is finished to the required depth. Etch rate of this process is 6 microns per minute. Figure 6.5 shows the schematic of Deep Reactive Ion Etching using Bosh process.

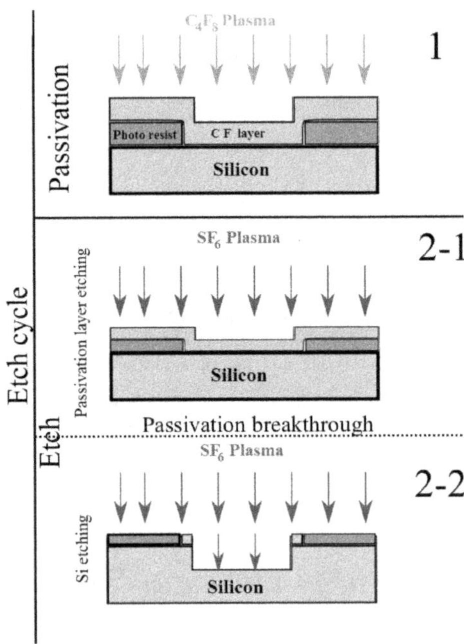

Figure 6.5: Schematic of Deep Reactive Ion Etching using Bosh process.

6.2.4   Cleaning

After the DRIE process, the etched sample is left with Photo-resist layer on the rear side and adhesive wax on the multilayers. Photo-resist layer can be completely removed by plasma ashing. Plasma ashing technique uses mono-atomic plasma

(Oxygen or Fluorine) to react with the photoresist and form ash which can be removed by evacuating the chamber. However, since the photoresist layer is on the non-reflective side of the mirror, we have not performed the plasma ashing but cleaned it with acetone which significantly removes the photo-resist layer. Wax is cleaned by heating the sample to $\sim 90^o$ C and clean with Isopropyl alcohol (IPA). Since the wax layer is directly on the multilayer structure, the removal of wax can probably disturb the multilayers. During the removal of wax, we have observed that the large period multilayers (d=5.5 nm) got significantly damaged. This is due to the poor adhesion of layers for large period multilayers. Figure 6.6 shows the photograph of the etched sample on the non-reflecting side of the multilayer mirror. Etch regions is a circle with a diameter of 5 mm.

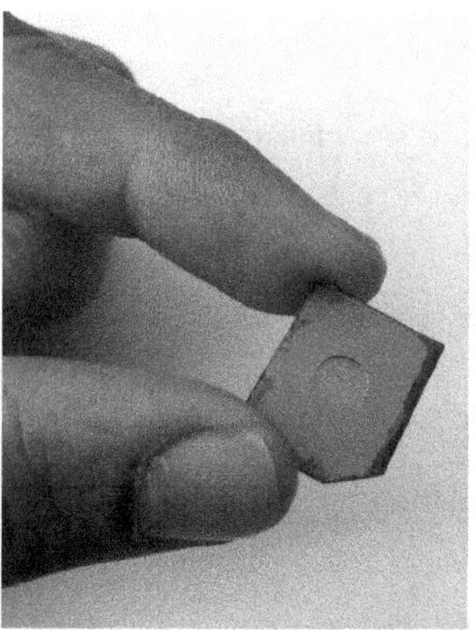

Figure 6.6: Photograph of the etched sample on the non-reflecting side of the multilayer mirror. Etch regions is a circle with a diameter of 5 mm.

6.3 Testing multilayer mirrors' reflectivity post Si etching

As explained earlier, the complete process of Si etching involves steps like heating the sample, applying and removing adhesive wax on multilayers and plasma etching the substrate. These steps can significantly alter the structural integrity of multilayers resulting the change in reflectivity. Residual wax leftover from cleaning process can form a contamination layer on the top surface which gives rise to oscillation in the reflectivity profile at small angles. Cleaning of wax can also peel of a few multilayers from the surface which results in the lowering of Bragg peak reflectivity. In-order to study the influence of etching process on the performance of multilayer mirrors, we have conducted X-ray reflectivity tests using 8.047 keV laboratory source on the mirrors and compared the results with the pre-etching reflectivity data.

We conducted etching on two mirrors with period 3.3 nm (d-3.3) and 5.4 nm (d-5.4). We observed that the reflectivity of the multilayer mirror of period 3.3 nm remained unchanged after the etching process. Figure 6.7 shows the comparison of the reflectivity profiles of the sample d-3.3 before and after etching process. The slight increase in the first Bragg peak reflectivity from 30% to 34% is due to change in the angular resolution of the refractometer. There is no trace of residual wax contamination layer on the top surface. But in the case of sample d-5.4 the Bragg peak reflectivity is significantly lowered from 20% to 5% after etching. Figure 6.8 shows the comparison of the reflectivity profiles of the sample d-5.4 before and after etching process. During the cleaning process, peel-off of few layers from the top surface is observed. This is due to low adhesion in the large period multilayer mirrors.

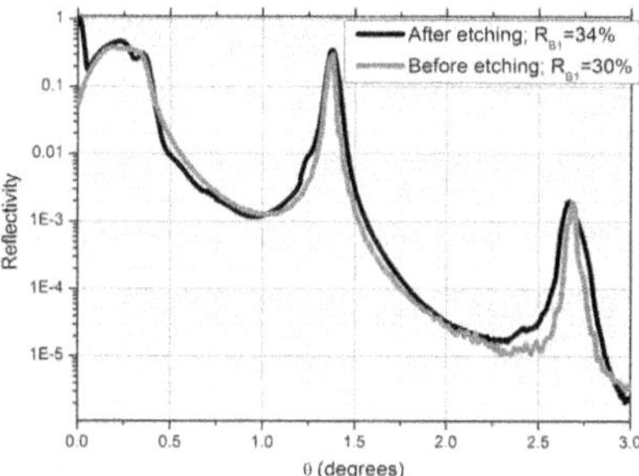

Figure 6.7: The comparison of the reflectivity profiles of the sample d-3.3 before and after etching process.

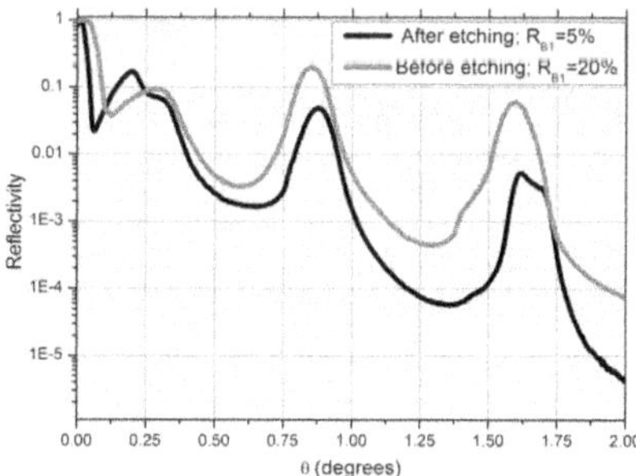

Figure 6.8: The comparison of the reflectivity profiles of the sample d-5.4 before and after etching process.

6.4 Estimation of X-ray transmission from the etched samples

We have conducted X-ray transmission measurements from the etched window of the samples to calculate absolute transmission and also to estimate the thickness of the substrate. X-ray transmission measurements are performed using 8.047

Table 6.1: The normal incidence 8.047 keV transmission efficiencies of two mirrors and two substrates along with the estimated substrate thickness at the etched region.

Sample ID	Transmission efficiency at 8.047 keV	Initial thickness of the substrate	After etching thickness
d-3.3	0.16	500 microns	129 ± 10 microns
d-5.4	0.16	500 microns	128 ± 10 microns
Si wafer 1	0.12	280 microns	148 ± 10 microns
Si wafer 2	0.13	280 microns	145 ± 10 microns

keV lab source by comparing the direct beam intensity to the transmitted beam intensity. Transmission efficiencies of two base 280 micron etched Si samples are measured along with the two multilayer mirrors. Table 6.1 shows the normal incidence 8.047 keV transmission efficiencies of two mirrors and two substrates along with the estimated substrate thickness at the etched region.

6.5 Summary

We performed Si etching using DRIE process on the non-reflecting side of the multilayer mirrors as well as bare silicon substrates. These mirrors are useful for developing hard X-ray transmission soft X-ray polarimeters using multilayer mirrors as a back-end instrument for a hard X-ray telescope. We observed that the etching process has significantly damaged the reflection efficiency of large period multilayer mirrors. However, short period multilayer mirrors (d $\sim$ 3 nm) are not affected by the etching process. These results are consistent with the earlier observations suggesting the high stability of short period multilayer mirrors over large periods. As described in chapter 5, soft X-ray polarimetry uses only short period multilayers (maximum period is 3.5 nm) for polarization measurements. Hence we have demonstrated Si etching of multilayer of short period multilayer mirrors as a reliable technique to develop ultra-thin substrate windows for increasing the hard X-ray transmission efficiency.

Chapter 7

X-ray telescope for the study of Solar Wind Charge eXchange reactions (SWCX)

7.1 Charge exchange reactions from the solar-system bodies

A stream of charged particles is being continuously released from the solar corona (outer atmosphere of the sun). These charged particles travel at supersonic speeds throughout the solar-system usually referred to as the Solar wind. Solar wind mostly consists of electrons, protons and alpha particles with kinetic energies ranging between 0.5-10 keV [Bame et al., 1968a], [Bame et al., 1968b], [Hundhausen, 1968], [Geiss et al., 1969]. Planets, their moons, and comets act like obstacles to the flow of solar-wind and often interacts via various mechanisms. Spreiter et. al in 1970 [Spreiter and Alksne, 1970] divided the solar-wind interaction into three different types: The Moon type, the Earth type, and the Venus type. This division is mainly classified on the presence of an atmosphere and/or a magnetic field.

The Moon-like bodies does not have either atmosphere or the magnetic field around them. The solar wind particles travel undisturbed until they impact the Lunar surface and then particles are absorbed and neutralized. Hence the Moon acts as a simple obstacle to the solar-wind and forms umbra and penumbra regions. In Moon-like bodies, solar wind interacts with the surface of the Moon. Figure 7.1 shows the schematic of the interaction of solar wind with Moon-like objects.

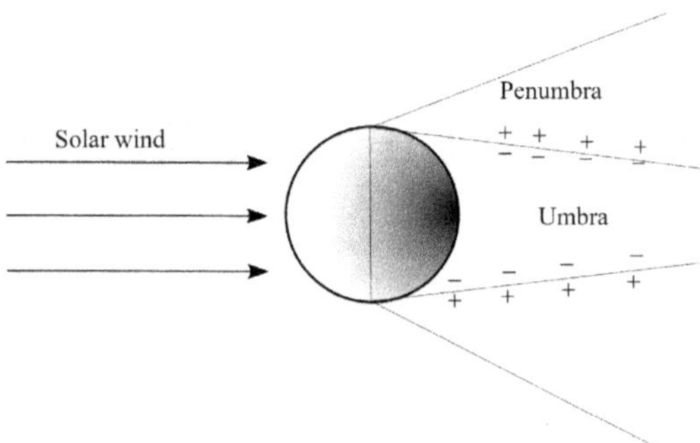

Figure 7.1: Schematic of the solar wind interaction with Moon-like objects with neither atmosphere nor magnetic field.

When objects have an intrinsic magnetic field like the Earth and the Jupiter, the interaction of the solar-wind particles (charged) is driven by the Lorentz force. The solar-wind magnetic field reconnects with the intrinsic magnetic field of the solar system body and a magnetosphere is often formed. The magnetosphere acts as an obstacle preventing the solar-wind from approaching too near to the object. Hence magnetic field of the objects acts as a protective shield from the solar wind. Figure 7.2 shows the schematic of the interaction of the solar wind with an Earth-like planet.

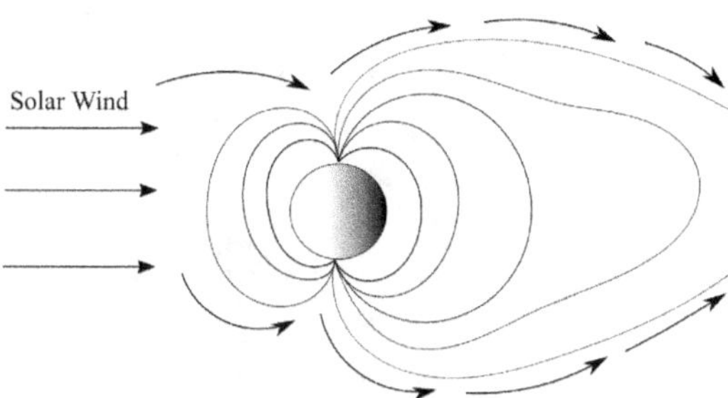

Figure 7.2: Schematic of the solar-wind interaction with the Earth like objects with magnetic field.

The intermediate case for the Moon like and Earth-like object is the Venus-like object. This category of objects do have a thick atmosphere but do not have a global magnetic field. Planets like Venus and Mars falls under this category. In this case, the solar wind directly interacts with the exosphere of the object and undergo charge exchange reactions. Schematic of the solar-wind interaction with the Venus-like objects is presented in figure 7.3.

Charge-exchange process The interaction between the solar wind plasma and the neutral planetary atmospheric gases is mainly due to charge exchange reactions [Elco, 1969]. In this process, the charge of the energetic plasma is exchanged with the neutral atom which ionises the neutral atom. The fundamental interaction between the energetic ion (A^+) and the atmospheric gas (G) is given by equation 7.1:

$$A^+ + G \rightarrow A + G^+ \tag{7.1}$$

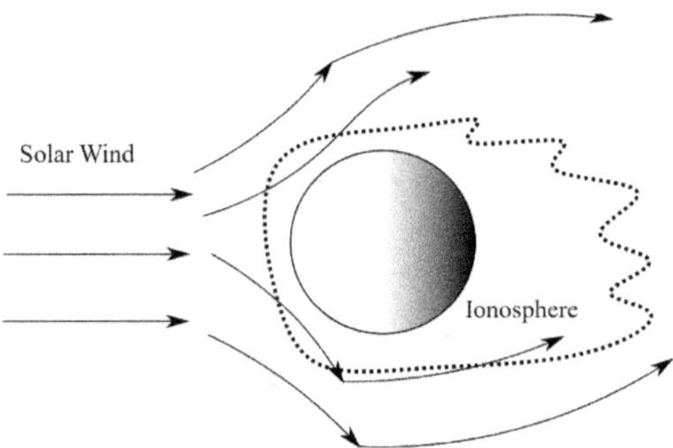

Figure 7.3: Schematic of the solar-wind interaction with the Venus like objects with thick atmosphere but no global magnetic field.

Some the examples of charge exchange reactions in the Mars and the Venus is given by [Kallio et al., 1997],

$$H^+_{solarwind} + H \rightarrow H_{soalrwind} + H^+ \tag{7.2}$$

$$H^+_{solarwind} + O \rightarrow H_{solarwind} + O^+ \tag{7.3}$$

Solar wind often consists of heavy multiply charged ions (example O^{6+}). The charge exchange reactions with multiply charged ions, say n times (A^{n+}) with neutral can result in production of photons (γ) 7.4 and 7.5.

$$A^{n+} + G \quad \rightarrow A^{*(n-1)+} + M^+ \tag{7.4}$$

$$\rightarrow A^{(n-1)+} + M^+ + \gamma \tag{7.5}$$

The superscript $*$ represents the excited state of the ion. The wavelength of the emitted photon is usually of the order 0.1- 1 keV [Kallio et al., 1997]. Hence X-ray observations can provide evidence for charge exchange reactions. Charge exchange is the fundamental process in atomic physics which has been studied in various contexts from a long time. X-ray observation of comets revealed the observational significance of this mechanism from solar system objects [Cravens, 2000], [Cravens and Maurellis, 2001], [Cravens, 2002], [Lisse, 2001], [Lisse et al., 1996] [Lisse et al., 1999], [Krasnopolsky et al., 2004], [Mumma et al., 1997] .

7.2 X-ray emission from Planets

The Sun is the brightest X-ray source in our solar system. X-ray emission from the Sun is mainly due to thermal emission from the million-degree hot coronal plasma. Planets do not have high surface temperatures to thermally produce X-rays. However, planets and moons can be X-ray bright either by scattering solar X-rays or by the X-ray fluorescence emission from the surface/ atmospheric atoms [Aikin, 1970]. Planetary bodies with an atmosphere can also produce X-rays via charge exchange reaction processes [Cravens, 2002], [Lisse et al., 2004]. Cometary X-ray studies from ROSAT X-ray instrument suggested that a similar mechanism should happen in other non-magnetic planets with atmosphere and produce X-rays [Dennerl et al., 1997]. X-ray observations of Venus and Mars have shown that the scattering occurs predominantly in the form of fluorescence on C, O and N atoms [Cravens and Maurellis, 2001], [Dennerl, 2008], [Bhardwaj et al., 2005a]. The atomic transitions which give rise to fluorescence are similar to the de-excitation process after charge exchange reactions. However, in the case of charge exchange, the atom is in a higher ionization state. Hence the binding energy of the inner shells is larger when compared to the case of fluorescence. Consequently, the X-ray energies resulting from charge exchange is slightly higher than the corresponding transitions from fluorescence [Bhardwaj et al., 2007]. This opens a possibility of spectrally separating emission from both processes.

The X-ray luminosity of the of the fluorescence X-rays depends on the solar X-ray flux and the X-ray luminosity due to charge exchange reaction depends on the velocity-density of solar winds. During the last few decades, X-ray emission from almost all solar system objects is observed. X-rays are observed from both polar and disk regions for magnetic planets like the Earth [Seward et al., 1976], [Petrosian et al., 1979], [Ezoe et al., 2014], Jupiter [Bell, 1980], [Metzger et al., 1980], [Metzger et al., 1983], [Barbosa, 1990], and the Saturn [Bhardwaj et al., 2005a], [Gilman et al., 1986], [Bhardwaj et al., 2005b], [Branduardi-Raymont et al., 2009]. X-rays from the Moon (Earth's moon) were observed by several satellites [Dolan, 1967], [Mandel'Shtam et al., 1968], [Michel, 1964], [Crawford et al., 2009], [Narendranath et al., 2010], [Narendranath et al., 2011] and confirmed the fluorescence X-ray emission from the lunar surface providing an excellent way to determine the elemental composition [Athiray et al., 2013]. First ever X-ray observation of the Moon was done by ROSAT in 1990 [Schmitt et al., 1991]. Figure 7.4 shows the X-ray image of the moon taken by the ROSAT satellite. X-ray emission from the day side of the Moon mostly arise by X-ray scattering and fluorescence. With advancements in the spectral resolution of X-ray instruments, the high-resolution spectroscopic observations of the Mars are conducted by the XMM-Newton telescope [Dennerl et al., 2006]. This study clearly indicated a clean separability of X-ray emission from charge exchange reactions and fluorescence. Figure 2.6 shows spectral imaging of Mars taken using XMM-Newton grating. Green and blue emission regions in Mars's exosphere are due to charge exchange reaction of Carbon and Oxygen respectively. X-ray emission shown in orange is due to fluorescence of solar X-rays on neutral Carbon and Oxygen. The X-ray observations from Venus are mainly limited due to small angular separation of Venus and Sun as viewed from the Earth's orbit. However, Chandra X-ray telescope could observe Venus confirming the X-ray line emissions from C, O and N [Dennerl et al., 2002]. These observations predicted that the X-ray emission from Venus is dominated by fluorescence. Figure 7.6 shows the first X-ray image of Venus taken by the Chandra X-ray telescope. Unlike in the case of the Moon, the fluorescent scattering in Venus is from the atmosphere and not from the surface.

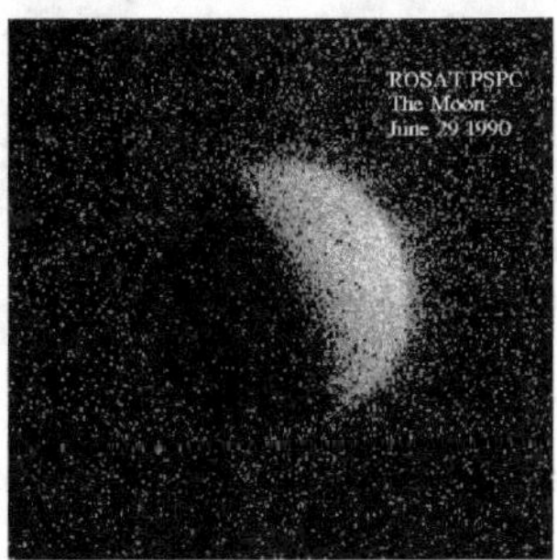

Figure 7.4: X-ray image from the Moon from ROSAT observations. Day side emission of the Moon is mainly due to scattering and fluorescent emission from the solar X-rays.

7.3 X-ray instrument for planetary observations

Despite the fact that X-ray observations of planetary bodies provide an excellent window to study many fundamental mechanisms occurring at planetary surfaces and atmosphere, the study is limited with insufficient observational data. General purpose X-ray instruments are not optimized for this application and hence it is difficult to establish the connection between predicted models and observations.

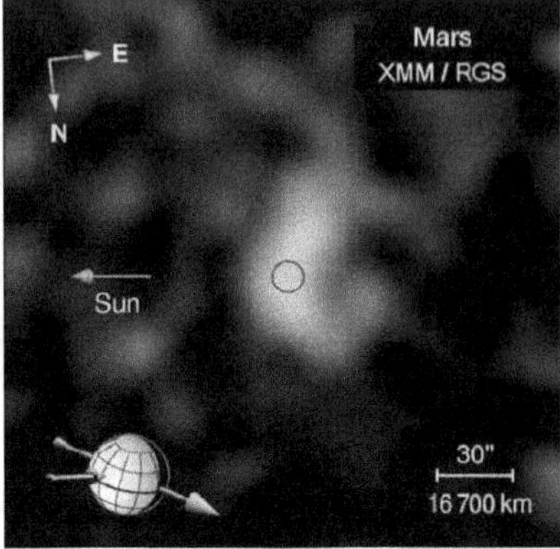

Figure 7.5: XMM-Newton observations of Mars. Green and blue emission is in the Mars' exosphere is due to charge exchange reaction of Carbon and Oxygen respectively. X-ray emission shown in orange is due to fluorescence of solar X-rays on neutral Carbon and Oxygen. Surface dimension of Mars is represented by the circle in the center.

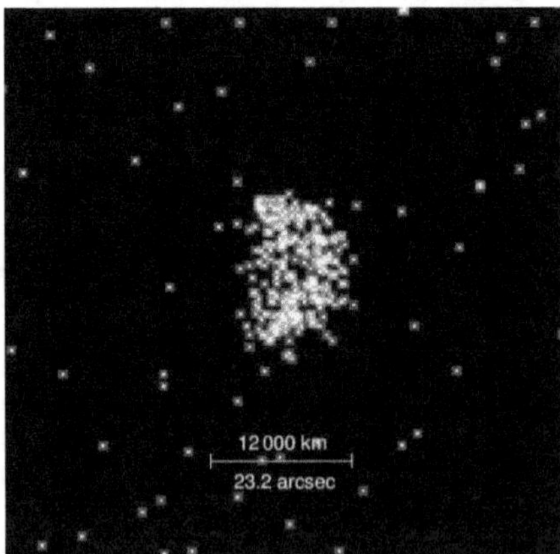

Figure 7.6: First X-ray image of Venus, obtained by the Chandra ACIS-I. The X-ray emission is mainly dominated by the fluorescence emission by neutral atoms in Venus' atmosphere by solar X-rays.

An X-ray instrument with good spatial and spectral resolution with good sensitivity of less than 1 keV orbiting the planetary body provides the perfect set of conditions to conduct the detailed study of these processes. To address this issue, we are working towards developing a soft X-ray telescope compatible for a planetary mission. This instrument aims to observe Venus-like planet with atmosphere but no magnetic field. X-ray flux from fluorescence and charge exchange reaction is usually low hence the major challenge of the X-ray telescope on an interplanetary mission is maintaining the trade-off between small size and large effective area.

To spectrally distinguish these two mechanisms, the instrument's spectral resolution should be better than 20 eV at 0.5 keV. X-ray detector's operating single pixel readouts cannot operate at such high resolutions. Additional back-end instruments like a grating increase the size and complexity of the instrument. However, the fluorescence and charge exchange reactions can be distinguished by the spatial. For non-magnetic planets, the fluorescence usually occurs at the lower atmosphere while the charge exchange reaction occurs at the exosphere which extends from 3 to 8 times the radius of the planet. Hence an eccentric orbit around the planet can probe different spatial regions of the planetary atmosphere which helps in spatially separating X-ray flux from fluorescence and charge exchange reactions.

7.3.1 Instrument design

The proposed instrument consists of a soft X-ray concentrator (to increase signal collection area) and a pixellated X-ray detector. The x-ray detector chosen is a back-illuminated CCD (Charge Coupled Device). The X-ray concentrator consists of single reflection grazing incidence mirrors optimized to reflect soft X-rays (<1 keV). Optics consists of 8 concentric shells of gold (Au)coated mirrors with a different angle of incidence to have a common focus. The maximum diameter of the concentrator is 20 cm and the focal length is 80 cm. The angle of incidence of the optics changes from 2.25^o to 3.53^o from inner shell to outer shell respectively. Overall active geometric area of the optics is $210cm^2$. Figure 7.7 shows the schematic of the instrument. Table 7.1 gives the specifications of all 8 shells of the concentrator.

Table 7.1: Specifications of all 8 shells of the X-ray concentrator.

Shell No.	Incidence angle	Diameter (cm)	Active area (cm^2)
1	2.25^o	13	16.1
2	2.4^o	13.8	18.3
3	2.56^o	14.7	20.8
4	2.73^o	15.7	23.6
5	2.91^o	16.8	26.8
6	3.11^o	17.8	30.5
7	3.31^o	19	34.7
8	3.53^o	20.3	39.4

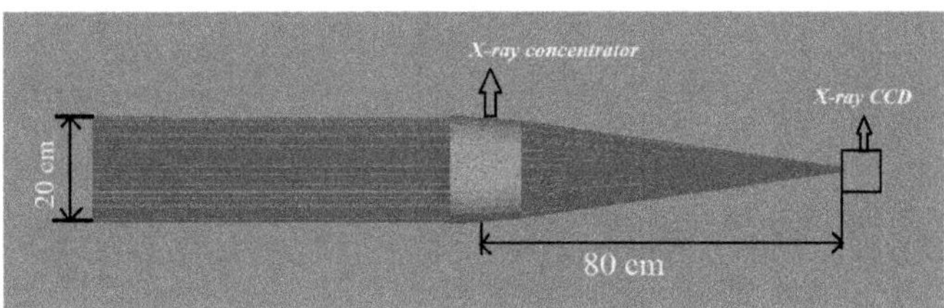

Figure 7.7: Schematic of the proposed instrument consist of an X-ray concentrator focussing X-rays on to a detector. Blue band indicates the X-rays light from the source.

7.3.2 Performance estimation of the optics

Since the X-ray concentrator consists of a single reflection conical shells, the off-axis PSF of the optics is severely limited by the Coma aberration. Hence the telescope is not suitable for imaging. However, the concentrator increases the signal to noise ratio of the observation by focusing X-rays on to the detector. Since angles of incidence of mirrors are different for different shells, the grazing incidence reflectivity varies significantly for different shells. Outer shells have larger angles and hence have low reflectivities. Figure 7.8 shows the reflectivity of all shells as a function of energy. The effective area of the telescope is estimated by multiplying the energy-dependent reflectivity to the effective geometric area of the shell. Effective geometric area contribution is higher for the outer shells as the radius and angle of incidence increases. Figure 7.9 shows the effective area contribution of all shells as a function of energy. The effective area decreases as the energy increases due to low reflectivity. The overall effective area of the optics is estimated by the sum of effective area contribution of all shells. Figure 7.10 shows the overall effective area of the optics.

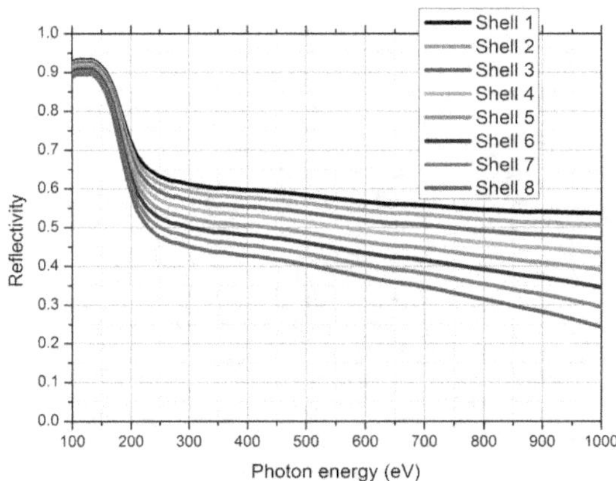

Figure 7.8: Reflectivity as a function of energy for all shells. Outer shells have have low reflectivity due to large angle of incidence.

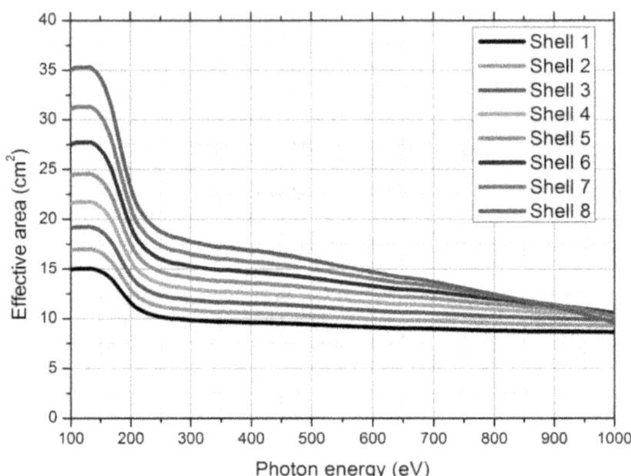

Figure 7.9: Effective area contribution of all shells as a function of energy. Outer shells have large effective area due to large radius of the shell and large angle of incidence.

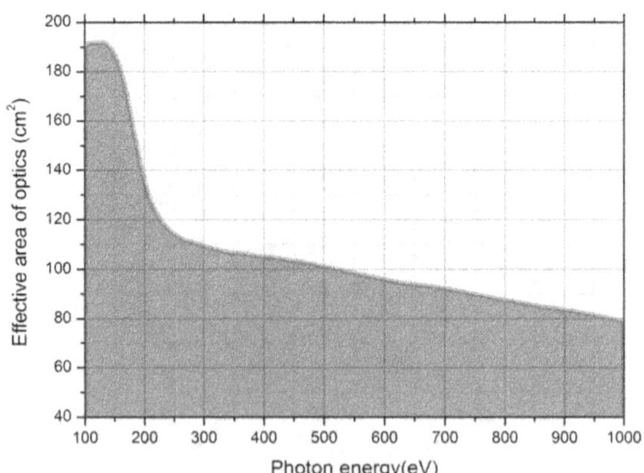

Figure 7.10: Overall effective of the optics as a function of energy. The effective area rapidly reduces as the photon energy increases.

7.3.3 Performance estimation of the instrument

Planetary bodies like Venus and Mars are very bright in visible light due to the reflection of solar light. The X-ray concentrator and the X-rays detector are also sensitive to visible light. Since the visible light flux is several orders of magnitude larger than the X-ray flux, an optical light blocking detector is placed in front of the detector. A 100 nm aluminium (Al) film acts as a good visible light blocking filter. However, this filter also attenuates X-rays mainly at soft X-ray region. The X-ray CCD also does not have 100% quantum efficiency throughout the spectrum. Figure 7.11 shows the quantum efficiency of the X-ray CCD along with the transmission efficiency of the 100 nm thick Al filter. Part (a) of the figure shows the quantum efficiency over the wide band. Part (b) shows the quantum efficiency over the region of interest for this instrument i.e. <1 keV.

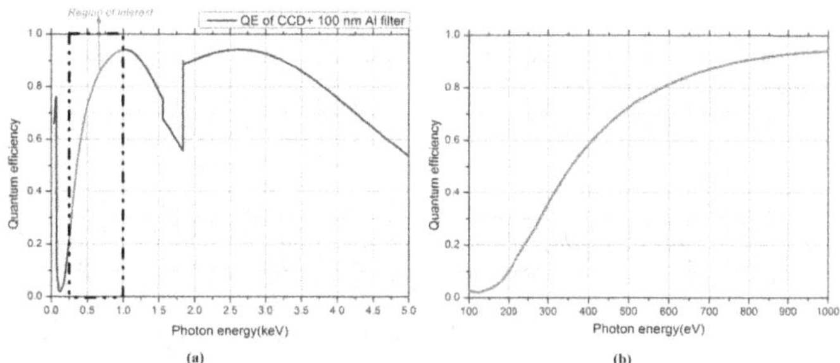

Figure 7.11: The quantum efficiency of the X-ray CCD along with the transmission efficiency of the 100 nm thick Al filter. (a) The quantum efficiency over the wide band. (b) The quantum efficiency over the region of interest for this instrument i.e. <1 keV.

The overall effective area of the instrument is estimated by convolving the quantum efficiency of the detector and filter with the effective area of the optics.

Figure 7.12 shows the estimated effective area of the entire instrument. The small effective area at low energies is mainly due to absorption of X-rays from the visible light blocking filter.

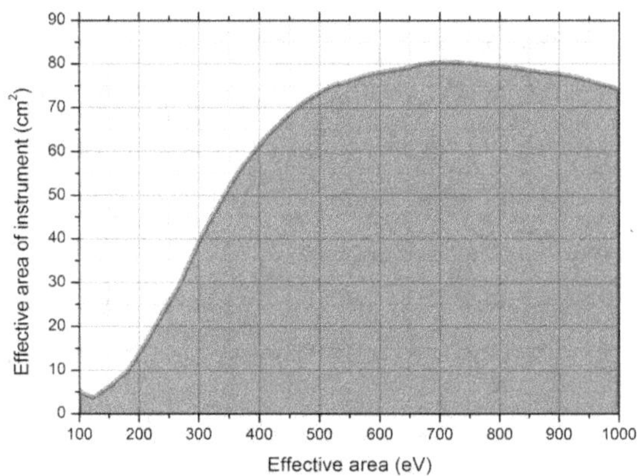

Figure 7.12: Estimated effective area of the entire instrument as a function of photon energy.

The instrument has an effective area over 70 cm^2 at 500 eV. This allows the instrument to conduct very sensitive observations over the entire atmosphere. We have conducted a simulation in Xspec [Arnaud, 1996] by feeding the response function of the instrument to the fake spectrum (user simulated spectrum to resemble the source spectral properties) of the source. We have considered a case of observing the Martian atmosphere using data available from earlier missions. Figure 7.13 shows the observed spectra of the Martian atmosphere by XMM-Newton telescope with a high-resolution spectrograph. X-ray emission is mostly by line emission with no significant continuum contribution. We have considered the brightest 14 line emissions arising either from fluorescence or charge exchange reactions. Figure

7.14 shows the fake line emissions estimated with different intensities (as per data
available from XMM-Newton) as input to the instrument. Figure 7.15 shows the
expected count rate from by the instrument. Several lines present in the atmospheric spectrum are very closely located spectrally. The spectral resolution of
the instrument is not sufficient to distinguish all the lines. However, by pointing
the instrument at various spatial positions in an elliptical orbit around the planet,
one can differentiate between the various line (Fluorescence lines from lower atmosphere and charge exchange lines from the upper atmosphere).

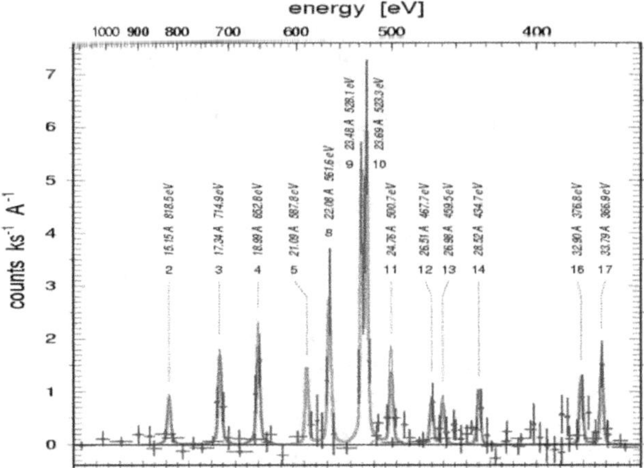

Figure 7.13: Observed X-ray spectra of the Mars by XMM-Newton telescope high
resolution spectrograph.

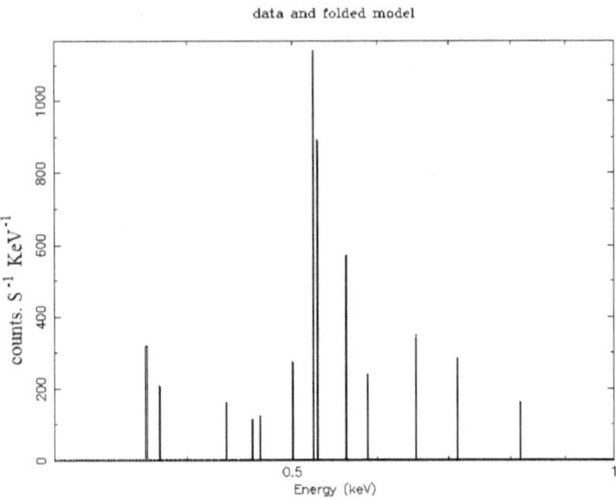

Figure 7.14: Fake spectra with several line emissions with respective intensities that was fed to the instrument response matrix in Xspec. These lines and intensities are taken from the observed flux from the Mars.

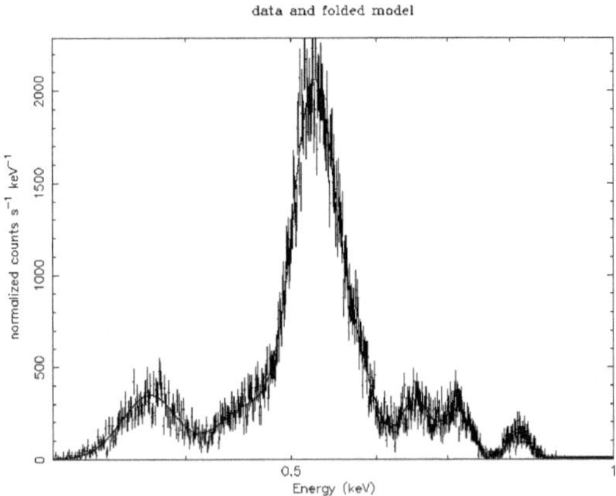

Figure 7.15: Expected count rate from the instrument when a spectra shown in figure 7.14 fed to the instrument response matrix.

7.4 Development and testing of the prototype X-ray concentrator

A prototype X-ray concentrator is developed using the spare X-ray mirrors from the previous Astrosat -SXT mission [Singh et al., 2017b]. Soft X-ray Telescope (SXT) mirrors are developed by depositing gold on the aluminium substrate using the replication process. These mirrors are originally made for 2-meter focal length double reflection optics. Since the currently proposed optics is a single reflection 80 cm concentrator, all mirror foils have to be reshaped accordingly. With the help of ISRO's R.R.Rao Satellite Center's (URSC) Apace Astronomy Group collaborators, we reshaped all mirror segments and developed a mechanical structure to hold the optics in the required geometry. The mechanical structure is completely 3-d printed using the facility available at URSC. The mechanical structure consists of a circular annulus with spider structure placed radially outwards either sides of the concentrator. Spider structure consists of groves with dimensions suitable for placing mirrors at required angles. The difference in the grove location between the front and the rare side of the optics provides the prescribed angle to a shell. Each mirror segment is a trapezium with a curvature on one axis to form a part of a circular ring. Figure 7.16 shows the photograph of the finished concentrator with X-ray mirrors assembled into the 3-d printed mechanical structure.

Preliminary testing of the mirror assembly is made by measuring the focusing properties of the optics. We have used a wide parallel beam optical light from the sun to get an initial estimate of the spot size at the focus. Imaging properties of this system significantly vary with the wavelength. It is difficult to estimate X-ray imaging properties by testing the optics at a visible wavelength. However, for a

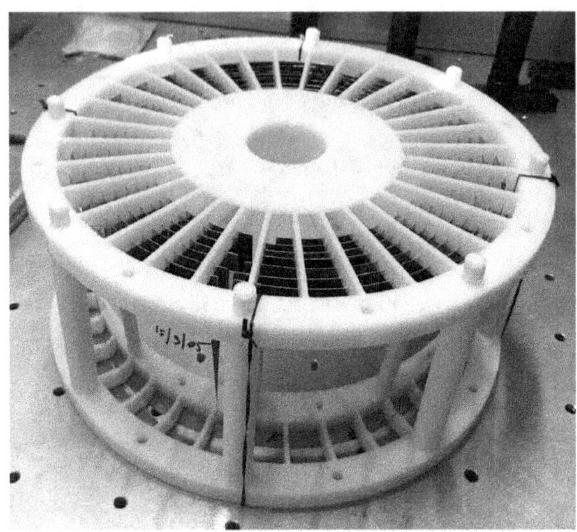

Figure 7.16: Photograph of the prototype X-ray concentrator developed using SXT spare mirrors. The mechanical structure in 3-d printed using URSC facility.

concentrator whose imaging property is not a major concern, visible light testing can give a fairly good approximate to the quality of the mirror alignment. We have used a Celostat system to track the sun and send the parallel beam sunlight constantly to the laboratory test bench. The X-ray concentrator is placed on an optical bench in the laboratory and a screen is placed at the focal plane of the optics. Schematic of the test setup of the calibration is shown in figure 7.17. Figure 7.18 shows the photograph of the test setup inside the laboratory showing sunlight illuminating the X-ray concentrator and a screen at the focus. Figure 7.19 shows the photograph of the spot at the focal plane screen of the concentrator. The spot size is approximately 0.4 cm for a concentrator of diameter 20 cm at a focal length of 80 cm. An initial estimate indicates that the concentration factor of 50 is achieved with this system which substantially increases the signal to noise ratio of the detection.

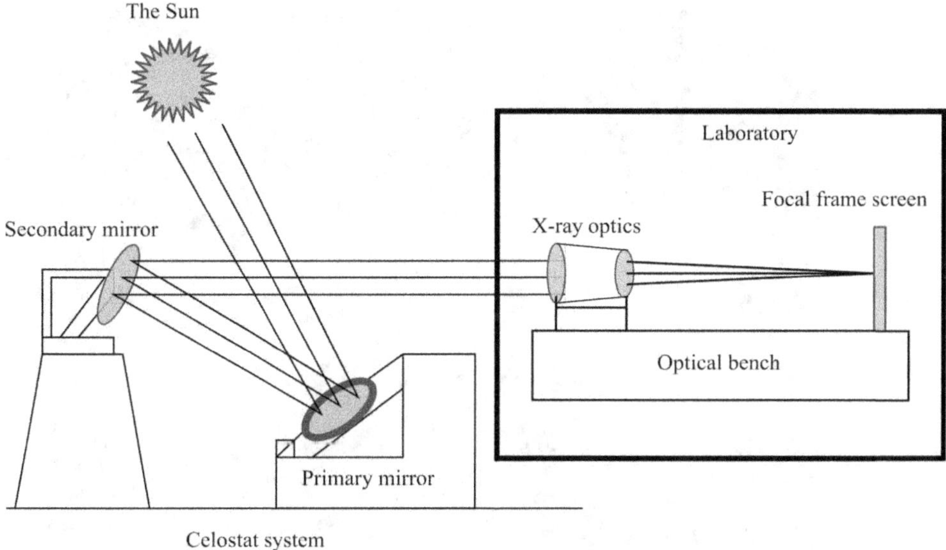

Figure 7.17: Schematic of the test setup used to calibrate the X-ray concentrator using the sunlight. A Celostat system is used continuously track the Sun to send parallel white light to feed the X-ray concentrator inside the laboratory.

7.5 Summary

In this chapter, we have presented an instrument design for observing the planetary atmosphere to study the charge exchange reactions from planetary exosphere as well as X-ray fluorescence emission measurement from the surface. The instrument consists of an X-ray concentrator with effective area on 80 cm^2 ideally suited to

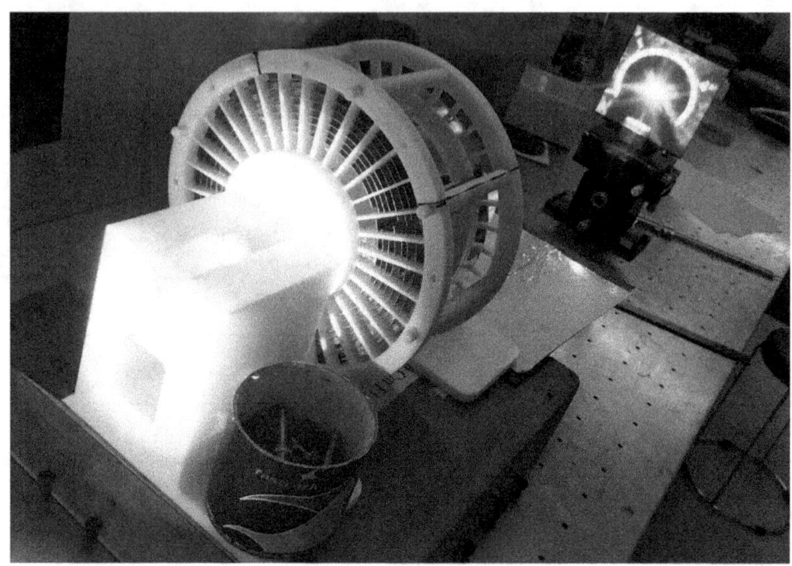

Figure 7.18: Photograph of the test setup in side the laboratory showing the sunlight illuminating the X-ray concentrator and a screen at the focus.

observe the Venus or the Mars from the planet's orbit. Short focal length of the instrument is ideally suited for a small payload for planetary mission. We have also assembled the prototype X-ray concentrator using spare mirrors from SXT-Astrosat and tested the focussing properties using optical white light source.

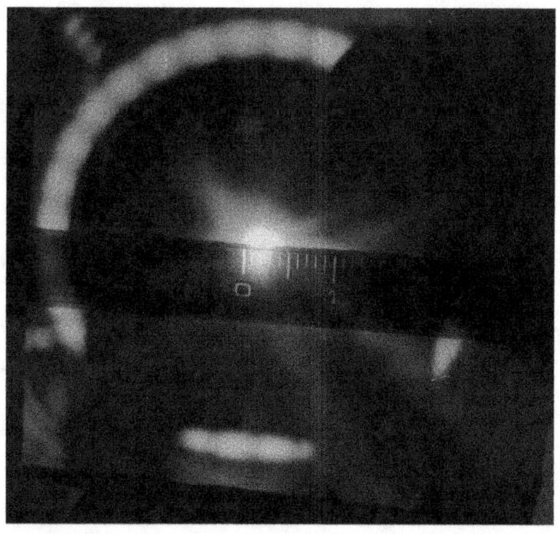

Figure 7.19: Photograph of the spot at the focal plane screen of the concentrator.

Chapter 8

Summary and future work

8.1 Major findings from the thesis work

1. High quality W/B_4C multilayer mirrors are fabricated with different design
   parameters like the number of bi-layers and period of bi-layers. All fabricated
   multilayer mirrors are characterized using multi-wavelength X-ray reflectivity
   analysis. We have studied the long time performance variations of multilayers
   over a span of 2 years. We have observed that the short period multilayers
   form a thick contamination layer on the top surface which results in the
   formation of oscillations in the reflectivity curve at lower angles. By imaging
   and spectroscopic studies of the mirror's surface, it is observed that the
   formation of contamination layer is due to oxidation of Tungsten layer in
   the mirror. Large thickness Boron-Carbide layer in large period multilayer
   mirrors prevents the Tungsten layer to interact with the atmospheric oxygen.
   These results are published in [Singam et al., 2018].

2. Performance stability of W/B_4C multilayer mirrors is studied by subjecting
   the mirrors to conditions similar to environmental conditions experienced
   by a satellite in low earth orbit. We have thermally cycled W/B_4C multi-

layer mirrors in the from -40° C to $+50^o$ C for several days in the profile analogues to the temperature variation expected in the low earth orbit. We have studied the performance and stability of these mirrors both before and after thermal cycling. We have observed that the short period multilayer mirrors are more stable to the dynamical thermal variations in the ambient temperature. We have observed reduction in reflectivity of multilayer mirrors with large period as well as observed the formation of wrinkles after thermal cycling the mirrors. We have studied the variation in residual stress in the multilayer mirrors due to thermal cycling. We have observed that the change in residual stress is large for large period multilayer mirrors. These results are published in [Singam et al., 2018]

3. A new design of a multilayer mirror based broad-band soft X-ray polarimeter is designed and its performance is estimated. This design uses a multilayer mirrors as polarization analysing mirrors at 45° to reflect only S-polarized X-rays. This instrument is capable of measuring the polarization of X-ray from 0.2-0.7 keV with a modulation factor more than 90°. Details of this instrument is published in [Panini et al., 2018].

4. We have successfully performed deep Si etching on the non reflecting surface of multilayer mirrors to increase the transmission efficiency of multilayer mirrors for hard X-rays. These mirrors are useful for developing an additional simultaneous back end soft X-ray polarimeter for a hard X-ray polarimeter. The major requirement of this arrangement is the development of thin substrate to transmit the hard X-rays (> 15 keV). Multilayer mirrors fabricated on the thick Si substrate (0.5 mm) absorbs hard X-rays which makes it difficult to design a configuration for the simultaneous observation of soft X-ray and hard X-ray polarimeter at a back end of a Hard X-ray telescope. Hence

we made a 5 mm, 0.1 mm thick substrate window by removing 0.4 mm of Si to make an aperture for for hard X-ray transmission.

5. A new, compact and a small size X-ray telescope is designed and proposed for studying the X-ray emission from planetary bodies. This instrument is having large sensitivity less than 1 keV to study fluorescence and charge exchange line emissions from the atmospheric atoms. Instrument consist of a grazing incidence X-ray optics and a focal plane detector at a focal length of 80 cm. A prototype X-ray concentrator system is developed with exact specifications is developed using Astrosat-SXT spare mirrors and focussing properties are calibrated using visible light. We have achieved a spot-size 5 mm by imaging the Sun in visible light.

8.2 Future work

8.2.1 Residual stress analysis of $W/B4C$ multilayer mirrors

By studying the stability of W/B_4C multilayer mirrors over thermal cycling, it is observed that the performance of large period multilayer mirrors forms prominent wrinkle structures on the layer structure. This can be related to the change in the residual stress of the mirror due to thermal cycling. We have measured the change in residual stress of the mirrors with two different periods and observed that the large period multilayer undergo larger change in residual stress than the short period mirrors. This phenomenon can be better understood by studying the evolution of residual stress on the substrate from the fabrication process and also by systematically conducting thermal cycling to all samples for different durations. This study gives the clear understanding of the origin and evolution of stress as a function of the period of bilayers both by intrinsic and extrinsic influences in

W/B_4C multilayer mirrors. This study also helps to develop stress mitigation techniques to use efficiently use W/B_4C multilayer mirrors for space applications.

8.2.2 Stability analysis of Si etched multilayer mirrors

This substrate multilayer mirrors are developed by etching the Si from the rare side of the mirror. Since these mirrors are sensitive to mechanical vibrations during the launch of the instrument to space. This thin substrate region of the mirror can become form pours as it undergoes large vibrations. This can also affect the structure of the multilayers which can lower the reflectivity. Chances of such accidents can be estimated by subjecting the mirrors to the vibrations analogous to the profile excepted during the take-off of a satellite launching vehicle. Stability of these mirrors to such conditions can be studied by microscopic imaging of the mirrors for identifying the pores formation and by X-ray reflectivity studies for quantifying the change multilayer structure of the mirror. Substrate etched mirrors can me more sensitive to the temperature variation of the surroundings. This is due the differential expansion/ contraction of the substrate material with respect to thin film. As the substrate is not uniform in the case of etched samples, the effect of thermal cycling can be different from the earlier studies of made of uniform thick substrate mirrors. Etched samples can form localized non-uniformities in the multilayer structures at the region where the substrate is etched. These effects can be systematically studied by conducting the thermal cycling to the etched samples and comparing the reflectivities of the mirrors before and after thermal cycling.

8.2.3 Development of active X-ray mirrors for high resolution X-ray imaging

Astronomical X-ray telescopes are severely limited by the optimized trade-off between the high resolution imaging and the large area optics. Effective area of the telescopes is enhanced by reducing the thickness of the mirror's substrate as it increases the packing density of the optics. Thin substrate X-ray mirrors also reduces the overall weight of the instrument. However, it is very difficult to develop and maintain the parabolic and hyperbolic figures in the mirrors developed by electro-forming or replication techniques. Hence X-ray mirrors developed by conical approximation are limited by the angular resolution.

Piezoelectric actuators

One the of the feasible techniques to address this problem is by developing the active X-ray mirrors. Active X-ray mirrors employee a mechanism to actively adjust the profile of the mirror to a required conic constant. The most popular technique to develop active X-ray mirrors is by developing Piezoelectric actuators on the rare side of the mirror. Piezoelectric materials like $Pb_{0.995}(Zr_{0.52}Ti_{0.48})_{0.99}Nb_{0.01}O_3$ is deposited on the non-reflecting side of the thin substrate and developed into several cells such that each cell acts as a micro actuator when applied voltage. Actuators exert a mechanical push on the mirror surface according to the applied voltage. By placing large number of actuators on the mirror, the shape and figure profiles of the mirrors can be changed in real time to achieve better spatial resolution from the telescope. Several optimization techniques have to be investigated from the coating of the piezoelectric layers to develop the fully functional actuator cells. As a part of future work, we work on the feasibility of developing and implementing piezoelectric actuators for on a prototype X-ray mirror.

Shape memory alloy substrates

High resolution X-ray mirrors can also be developed by using shape memory alloy substrates like TiNi for mirrors. Shape memory alloys can be originally made into the shape suitable for the high resolution X-ray optics. When the original shape is deformed during the launch or overtime, the initial shape can be retained by heating the substrate. Shape memory alloys are demonstrated in several actuator applications in medical, aircraft and auto-mobile applications. This technique do not allow real time profile modifications to the mirror but it can retain its original shape obtained during the processing phase. Feasibility study of using different shape memory alloys as a substrate materials for X-ray mirrors will be studied further.

8.3   Conclusion

As described in this thesis, our progress in understanding the behaviour of multilayer mirrors helps in developing several next-generation astronomical X-ray instruments with enhanced capabilities. Multilayer mirrors help in improving the current limitations of X-ray instruments by increasing the numerical aperture of soft X-ray telescopes as well as by improving the bandwidth of operation towards hard X-rays. Multilayer mirrors also contribute in opening a completely new window of observing the universe such as soft X-ray polarimetry. Capacity to fabricate a variety of good quality multilayer mirrors has reinvigorate new possibilities in the otherwise saturating field of astronomical X-ray optics.

Bibliography

[Ables, 1968] Ables, J. G. (1968). Fourier transform photography: a new method for X-ray astronomy. *Proceedings of the Astronomical Society of Australia*, 1:172.

[Aikin, 1970] Aikin, A. C. (1970). X-Ray Glow from Planetary Atmospheres. *Nature*, 227:1334.

[Aitken, 1968] Aitken, D. W. (1968). Recent Advances in X-Ray Detection Technology. *IEEE Transactions on Nuclear Science*, 15:10–46.

[Almeida and Pillet, 1993] Almeida, J. S. and Pillet, V. M. (1993). Polarizing properties of grazing-incidence x-ray mirrors - comment. *ao*.

[Angel et al., 1969] Angel, J. R., Novick, R., vanden Bout, P., and Wolff, R. (1969). Search for X-Ray Polarization in Sco X-1. *Physical Review Letters*, 22:861–865.

[Arefiev et al., 2008] Arefiev, V., Pavlinsky, M., Lapshov, I., Tkachenko, A., Sazonov, S., Revnivtsev, M., Semena, N., Buntov, M., Vikhlinin, A., Gubarev, M., O'Dell, S., Ramsey, B., Romaine, S., Swartz, D., Weisskopf, M., Hasinger, G., Predehl, P., Grigorovich, S., Litvin, D., Meidinger, N., and Strüder, L. W. (2008). ART-XC: a medium-energy x-ray telescope system for the Spectrum-R-Gamma mission. In *Space Telescopes and Instrumentation 2008: Ultraviolet to Gamma Ray*, volume 7011 of *Society of Photo-Optical Instrumentation Engineers (SPIE) Conference Series*, page 70110L.

[Arnaud, 1996] Arnaud, K. A. (1996). XSPEC: The First Ten Years. In Jacoby, G. H. and Barnes, J., editors, *Astronomical Data Analysis Software and Systems V*, volume 101 of *Astronomical Society of the Pacific Conference Series*, page 17.

[Athiray et al., 2013] Athiray, P. S., Narendranath, S., Sreekumar, P., Dash, S. K., and Babu, B. R. S. (2013). Validation of methodology to derive elemental abundances from X-ray observations on Chandrayaan-1. *Planetary and Space Science*, 75:188–194.

[Athiray et al., 2014] Athiray, P. S., Narendranath, S., Sreekumar, P., and Grande, M. (2014). C1XS results-First measurement of enhanced sodium on the lunar surface. *Planetary and Space Science*, 104:279–287.

[Atwood et al., 2009] Atwood, W. B., Abdo, A. A., Ackermann, M., Althouse, W., Anderson, B., Axelsson, M., Baldini, L., Ballet, J., Band, D. L., Barbiellini, G., Bartelt, J., Bastieri, D., Baughman, B. M., Bechtol, K., Bdrde, D., Bellardi, F., Bellazzini, R., Berenji, B., Bignami, G. F., Bisello, D., Bissaldi, E., Blandford, R. D., Bloom, E. D., Bogart, J. R., Bonamente, E., Bonnell, J., Borgland, A. W., Bouvier, A., Bregeon, J., Brez, A., Brigida, M., Bruel, P., Burnett, T. H., Busetto, G., Caliandro, G. A., Cameron, R. A., Caraveo, P. A., Carius, S., Carlson, P., Casandjian, J. M., Cavazzuti, E., Ceccanti, M., Cecchi, C., Charles, E., Chekhtman, A., Cheung, C. C., Chiang, J., Chipaux, R., Cillis, A. N., Ciprini, S., Claus, R., Cohen-Tanugi, J., Condamoor, S., Conrad, J., Corbet, R., Corucci, L., Costamante, L., Cutini, S., Davis, D. S., Decotigny, D., DeKlotz, M., Dermer, C. D., de Angelis, A., Digel, S. W., do Couto e Silva, E., Drell, P. S., Dubois, R., Dumora, D., Edmonds, Y., Fabiani, D., Farnier, C., Favuzzi, C., Flath, D. L., Fleury, P., Focke, W. B., Funk, S., Fusco, P.,

Gargano, F., Gasparrini, D., Gehrels, N., Gentit, F.-X., Germani, S., Giebels, B., Giglietto, N., Giommi, P., Giordano, F., Glanzman, T., Godfrey, G., Grenier, I. A., Grondin, M.-H., Grove, J. E., Guillemot, L., Guiriec, S., Haller, G., Harding, A. K., Hart, P. A., Hays, E., Healey, S. E., Hirayama, M., Hjalmarsdotter, L., Horn, R., Hughes, R. E., Jhannesson, G., Johansson, G., Johnson, A. S., Johnson, R. P., Johnson, T. J., Johnson, W. N., Kamae, T., Katagiri, H., Kataoka, J., Kavelaars, A., Kawai, N., Kelly, H., Kerr, M., Klamra, W., Kndlseder, J., Kocian, M. L., Komin, N., Kuehn, F., Kuss, M., Landriu, D., Latronico, L., Lee, B., Lee, S.-H., Lemoine-Goumard, M., Lionetto, A. M., Longo, F., Loparco, F., Lott, B., Lovellette, M. N., Lubrano, P., Madejski, G. M., Makeev, A., Marangelli, B., Massai, M. M., Mazziotta, M. N., McEnery, J. E., Menon, N., Meurer, C., Michelson, P. F., Minuti, M., Mirizzi, N., Mitthumsiri, W., Mizuno, T., Moiseev, A. A., Monte, C., Monzani, M. E., Moretti, E., Morselli, A., Moskalenko, I. V., Murgia, S., Nakamori, T., Nishino, S., Nolan, P. L., Norris, J. P., Nuss, E., Ohno, M., Ohsugi, T., Omodei, N., Orlando, E., Ormes, J. F., Paccagnella, A., Paneque, D., Panetta, J. H., Parent, D., Pearce, M., Pepe, M., Perazzo, A., Pesce-Rollins, M., Picozza, P., Pieri, L., Pinchera, M., Piron, F., Porter, T. A., Poupard, L., Rain, S., Rando, R., Rapposelli, E., Razzano, M., Reimer, A., Reimer, O., Reposeur, T., Reyes, L. C., Ritz, S., Rochester, L. S., Rodriguez, A. Y., Romani, R. W., Roth, M., Russell, J. J., Ryde, F., Sabatini, S., Sadrozinski, H. F.-W., Sanchez, D., Sander, A., Sapozhnikov, L., Parkinson, P. M. S., Scargle, J. D., Schalk, T. L., Scolieri, G., Sgr, C., Share, G. H., Shaw, M., Shimokawabe, T., Shrader, C., Sierpowska-Bartosik, A., Siskind, E. J., Smith, D. A., Smith, P. D., Spandre, G., Spinelli, P., Starck, J.-L., Stephens, T. E., Strickman, M. S., Strong, A. W., Suson, D. J., Tajima, H., Takahashi, H., Takahashi, T., Tanaka, T., Tenze, A., Tether, S., Thayer, J. B., Thayer, J. G., Thompson, D. J., Tibaldo, L., Tibolla, O., Torres, D. F.,

Tosti, G., Tramacere, A., Turri, M., Usher, T. L., Vilchez, N., Vitale, V., Wang, P., Watters, K., Winer, B. L., Wood, K. S., Ylinen, T., and Ziegler, M. (2009). The large area telescope on the fermi gamma-ray space telescope mission. *The Astrophysical Journal*, 697(2):1071.

[Audard et al., 2001] Audard, M., Behar, E., Güdel, M., Raassen, A. J. J., Porquet, D., Mewe, R., Foley, C. R., and Bromage, G. E. (2001). The XMM-Newton view of stellar coronae: High-resolution X-ray spectroscopy of Capella. *Astron. Astrophys.*, 365:L329–L335.

[Auger, 1926] Auger, P. (1926). Leffet photoelectrique compose. *Annales de Physique*, 10:183–253.

[Ballet and Decourchelle, 2002] Ballet, J. and Decourchelle, A. (2002). X-ray spectroscopy of supernova remnants. *New Astronomy Reviews*, 46:507–511.

[Bame et al., 1968a] Bame, S. J., Hundhausen, A. J., Asbridge, J. R., and Strong, I. B. (1968a). Ion Composition of the Solar Wind. *The Astronomical Journal Supplement*, 73:55.

[Bame et al., 1968b] Bame, S. J., Hundhausen, A. J., Asbridge, J. R., and Strong, I. B. (1968b). Solar Wind Ion Composition. *Physical Review Letters*, 20:393–395.

[Barbosa, 1990] Barbosa, D. D. (1990). Bremsstrahlung X rays from Jovian auroral electrons. *Journal of Geophysical Research*, 95:14969–14976.

[Baring, 2008] Baring, M. G. (2008). Photon Splitting and Pair Conversion in Strong Magnetic Fields. In Dubois, D. M., editor, *American Institute of Physics Conference Series*, volume 1051 of *American Institute of Physics Conference Series*, pages 53–64.

[Bass et al., 2010] Bass, M., DeCusatis, C., Enoch, J., Lakshminarayanan, V., Li, G., Macdonald, C., Mahajan, V., and Van Stryland, E. (2010). *Handbook of Optics, Second Edition Volume III: Design, Fabrication and Testing, Sources and Detectors, Radiometry and Photometry.* McGraw-Hill, Inc., New York, NY, USA, 3 edition.

[Bell, 1980] Bell, P. M. (1980). X-Rays detected from Jupiter. *EOS Transactions*, 61:537–537.

[Bhardwaj et al., 2005a] Bhardwaj, A., Elsner, R., Gladstone, R., Cravens, T., Waite, H., Branduardi-Raymont, G., Ostgaard, N., Dennerl, K., Lisse, C., Kharchenko, V., Hoekstra, R., and Beiersdorfer, P. (2005a). A Comparative View of X-rays from the Solar System. In *AGU Spring Meeting Abstracts*, volume 2005, pages P43A–05.

[Bhardwaj et al., 2007] Bhardwaj, A., Elsner, R. F., Randall Gladstone, G., Cravens, T. E., Lisse, C. M., Dennerl, K., Branduardi-Raymont, G., Wargelin, B. J., Hunter Waite, J., Robertson, I., Østgaard, N., Beiersdorfer, P., Snowden, S. L., and Kharchenko, V. (2007). X-rays from solar system objects. *Planetary Space Science*, 55:1135–1189.

[Bhardwaj et al., 2005b] Bhardwaj, A., Elsner, R. F., Waite, J. Hunter, J., Gladstone, G. R., Cravens, T. E., and Ford, P. G. (2005b). Chandra Observation of an X-Ray Flare at Saturn: Evidence of Direct Solar Control on Saturn's Disk X-Ray Emissions. *Astrophys. J.*, 624:L121–L124.

[Bisnovatyi-Kogan and Fridman, 1969] Bisnovatyi-Kogan, G. S. and Fridman, A. M. (1969). A Mechanism for Emission of X Rays by a Neutron Star. *Astronomicheskii Zhurnal*, 46:721.

[Black et al., 2007] Black, J. K., Baker, R. G., Deines-Jones, P., Hill, J. E., and Jahoda, K. (2007). X-ray polarimetry with a micropattern TPC. *Nuclear Instruments and Methods in Physics Research A*, 581:755–760.

[Borkowski and Kopp, 1972] Borkowski, C. J. and Kopp, M. K. (1972). Proportional Counter Photon Camera. *IEEE Transactions on Nuclear Science*, 19:161–168.

[Born and Wolf, 1975] Born, M. and Wolf, E. (1975). *Principles of optics. Electromagnetic theory of propagation, interference and diffraction of light.*

[Boyle and Smith, 1970] Boyle, W. S. and Smith, G. E. (1970). Charge coupled semiconductor devices. *The Bell System Technical Journal*, 49(4):587–593.

[Bradt et al., 1993] Bradt, H. V., Rothschild, R. E., and Swank, J. H. (1993). X-ray timing explorer mission. *Astron. Astrophys. Suppl.*, 97:355–360.

[Branduardi-Raymont, 2011] Branduardi-Raymont, G. (2011). High Resolution X-ray Views of Solar System Objects. In *American Astronomical Society Meeting Abstracts #218*, volume 218 of *American Astronomical Society Meeting Abstracts*, page 102.02.

[Branduardi-Raymont et al., 2009] Branduardi-Raymont, G., Bjardwaj, A., Elsner, R. F., Gladstone, G. R., Rodriguez, P., Waite, J. H., and Cravens, T. E. (2009). X-rays from Saturn: A study with XMM-Newton and Chandra. In *European Planetary Science Congress 2009*, page 576.

[Brewster, 1815] Brewster, D. (1815). On the Law of the Partial Polarization of Light by Reflexion. [Abstract]. *Proceedings of the Royal Society of London Series I*, 2:387–389.

[Cameron, 1959] Cameron, A. G. (1959). Neutron Star Models. *Astrophys. J.*, 130:884.

[Canizares, 1987] Canizares, C. R. (1987). X-Rays from Galaxies and Clusters of Galaxies - Observations and Phenomenology. In Kormendy, J. and Knapp, G. R., editors, *Dark matter in the universe*, volume 117 of *IAU Symposium*, page 165.

[Chauvin et al., 2018] Chauvin, M., Florén, H. G., Friis, M., Jackson, M., Kamae, T., Kataoka, J., Kawano, T., Kiss, M., Mikhalev, V., Mizuno, T., Tajima, H., Takahashi, H., Uchida, N., and Pearce, M. (2018). The PoGO+ view on Crab off-pulse hard X-ray polarization. *Mon. Not. Roy. Astron. Soc.*, 477:L45–L49.

[Cheung, 2004] Cheung, C. C. (2004). *Studies of the kilo-parsec scale radio and optical emission from X-ray jets in active galactic nuclei*. PhD thesis, BRANDEIS UNIVERSITY.

[Christensen et al., 1995] Christensen, F. E., Joensen, K. D., Gorenstein, P., Priedhorsky, W. C., Westergaard, N. J., and Schnopper, H. W. (1995). A Hard X-Ray Telescope/Concentrator Design Based on Graded Period Multilayer Coatings. *Experimental Astronomy*, 6:33–46.

[Cline et al., 1968] Cline, T. L., Holt, S. S., and Hones, E. W., J. (1968). High-energy X rays from the solar flare of July 7, 1966. *Journal of Geophysical Research*, 73:434.

[Colgate, 1968] Colgate, S. A. (1968). Prompt gamma rays and X-rays from supernovae. *Canadian Journal of Physics*, 46:S476–S480.

[Compton, 1923] Compton, A. H. (1923). A Quantum Theory of the Scattering of X-rays by Light Elements. *Physical Review*, 21:483–502.

[Costa et al., 1997] Costa, E., Frontera, F., Heise, J., Feroci, M., in't Zand, J., Fiore, F., Cinti, M. N., Dal Fiume, D., Nicastro, L., Orlandini, M., Palazzi, E., Rapisarda#, M., Zavattini, G., Jager, R., Parmar, A., Owens, A., Molendi, S., Cusumano, G., Maccarone, M. C., Giarrusso, S., Coletta, A., Antonelli, L. A., Giommi, P., Muller, J. M., Piro, L., and Butler, R. C. (1997). Discovery of an X-ray afterglow associated with the γ-ray burst of 28 February 1997. *Nature*, 387:783–785.

[Costa et al., 2001] Costa, E., Soffitta, P., Bellazzini, R., Brez, A., Lumb, N., and Spandre, G. (2001). An efficient photoelectric X-ray polarimeter for the study of black holes and neutron stars. *Nature*, 411:662–665.

[Cravens, 2000] Cravens, T. (2000). X-ray emission from comets and planets. *Advances in Space Research*, 26(10):1443 – 1451. Planetary Ionospheres and Magnetospheres.

[Cravens, 2002] Cravens, T. E. (2002). X-ray Emission from Comets. *Science*, 296:1042–1046.

[Cravens and Maurellis, 2001] Cravens, T. E. and Maurellis, A. N. (2001). X-ray emission from scattering and fluorescence of solar X-rays at Venus and Mars. *Geophysical Research Letters*, 28:3043–3046.

[Crawford et al., 2009] Crawford, I. A., Kellett, B. J., Grande, M., Maddison, B. J., Howe, C. J., Swinyard, B., Joy, K. H., Sreekumar, P., Narendranath, S., Huovelin, J., and C1XS Science Team (2009). First results from the C1XS X-ray spectrometer on board Chandrayaan-1. *Geochimica et Cosmochimica Acta Supplement*, 73:A250.

[Dennerl, 2003] Dennerl, K. (2003). Discovery of X-rays from Mars with Chandra. *Astronomische Nachrichten Supplement*, 324:28.

[Dennerl, 2008] Dennerl, K. (2008). X-rays from Venus observed with Chandra. *Planetary and Space Science*, 56:1414–1423.

[Dennerl et al., 2002] Dennerl, K., Burwitz, V., Englhauser, J., Lisse, C., and Wolk, S. (2002). Discovery of X-rays from Venus with Chandra. *Astron. Astrophys.*, 386:319–330.

[Dennerl et al., 1997] Dennerl, K., Englhauser, J., and Trümper, J. (1997). X-ray emissions from comets detected in the Rontgen X-ray satellite all-sky survey. *Science*, 277:1625–1630.

[Dennerl et al., 2006] Dennerl, K., Lisse, C. M., Bhardwaj, A., Burwitz, V., Englhauser, J., Gunell, H., Holmström, M., Jansen, F., Kharchenko, V., and Rodríguez- Pascual, P. M. (2006). First observation of Mars with XMM-Newton. High resolution X-ray spectroscopy with RGS. *Astron. Astrophys.*, 451:709–722.

[Dicke, 1968] Dicke, R. H. (1968). Scatter-Hole Cameras for X-Rays and Gamma Rays. *Astrophys. J.*, 153:L101.

[Dolan, 1967] Dolan, J. F. (1967). Lunar x-ray fluorescence excited by Solar x-radiation. *Astron. J.*, 72:297.

[Doschek, 1990] Doschek, G. A. (1990). Soft X-ray spectroscopy of solar flares - an overview. *Astrophys. J.S*, 73:117–130.

[Dovciak et al., 2008] Dovciak, M., Muleri, F., Goosmann, R. W., Karas, V., and Matt, G. (2008). Thermal disc emission from a rotating black hole: X-ray polarization signatures. *Mon. Not. Roy. Astron. Soc.*, 391:32–38.

[Doxsey, 1975] Doxsey, R. (1975). Positions of X-Ray Sources. *International Astronomical Union Circular*, 2820:1.

[Dubner et al., 2017] Dubner, G., Castelletti, G., Kargaltsev, O., Pavlov, G. G., Bietenholz, M., and Talavera, A. (2017). Morphological Properties of the Crab Nebula: A Detailed Multiwavelength Study Based on New VLA, HST, Chandra, and XMM-Newton Images. *Astrophys. J.*, 840:82.

[Duncan and Thompson, 1992] Duncan, R. C. and Thompson, C. (1992). Formation of Very Strongly Magnetized Neutron Stars: Implications for Gamma-Ray Bursts. *Astrophys. J.*, 392:L9.

[Elco, 1969] Elco, R. A. (1969). Interaction of the solar wind with planetary atmospheres. *Journal of Geophysical Research*, 74:5073.

[Evans et al., 1988] Evans, B. L., Al-Dabbagh, J., and Kent, B. J. (1988). The Soft X-Ray To Euv Performance Of Plane And Concave Pt-Si Multilayer Mirrors. In Christensen, F. E., editor, *X-ray multilayers for diffractometers, monochromators, and spectrometers*, volume 984 of *Society of Photo-Optical Instrumentation Engineers (SPIE) Conference Series*, pages 104–110.

[Evans et al., 1989] Evans, B. L., Al-Dabbagh, J., and Kent, B. J. (1989). The soft X-ray to EUV performance of plane and concave Pt-Si multilayer mirrors. *Journal of Modern Optics*, 36:471–481.

[Ezoe et al., 2014] Ezoe, Y., Ishisaki, Y., Ohashi, T., Mitsuishi, I., Ishikawa, K., Miyoshi, Y., Fujimoto, R., Kasahara, S., Kimura, T., Hasegawa, H., Fujimoto, M., Mitsuda, K., Nishijo, K., and Noda, A. (2014). Suzaku observations of diffuse X-rays from the Earth's magnetosphere and beyond. In Ishida, M., Petre, R., and Mitsuda, K., editors, *Suzaku-MAXI 2014: Expanding the Frontiers of the X-ray Universe*, page 39.

[Franceschini et al., 1994] Franceschini, A., La Franca, F., Cristiani, S., and Martin- Mirones, J. M. (1994). X-ray versus Optically Selected Active Galactic Nuclei: A Comparative Study of the Luminosity Functions and Evolution Rates. *Mon. Not. Roy. Astron. Soc.*, 269:683.

[Freund and Suresh, 2004] Freund, L. B. and Suresh, S. (2004). *Thin Film Materials: Stress, Defect Formation and Surface Evolution*. Cambridge University Press.

[Frost, 1969] Frost, K. J. (1969). Rapid Fine Structure in a Burst of Hard Solar X-Rays Observed by OSO-5. *Astrophys. J. Lett.*, 158:L159.

[Geiss et al., 1969] Geiss, J., Eberhardt, P., Signer, P., Buehler, F., and Meister, J. (1969). *The Solar-Wind Composition Experiment*, page 183.

[Giacconi et al., 1979] Giacconi, R., Branduardi, G., Briel, U., Epstein, A., Fabricant, D., Feigelson, E., Forman, W., Gorenstein, P., Grindlay, J., Gursky, H., Harnden, F. R., Henry, J. P., Jones, C., Kellogg, E., Koch, D., Murray, S., Schreier, E., Seward, F., Tananbaum, H., Topka, K., Van Speybroeck, L., Holt, S. S., Becker, R. H., Boldt, E. A., Serlemitsos, P. J., Clark, G., Canizares, C., Markert, T., Novick, R., Helfand, D., and Long, K. (1979). The Einstein (HEAO 2) X-ray Observatory. *Astrophys. J.*, 230:540–550.

[Giacconi et al., 1962] Giacconi, R., Gursky, H., Paolini, F. R., and Rossi, B. B. (1962). Evidence for x rays from sources outside the solar system. *Phys. Rev. Lett.*, 9:439–443.

[Giacconi et al., 1971] Giacconi, R., Kellogg, E., Gorenstein, P., Gursky, H., and Tananbaum, H. (1971). An X-Ray Scan of the Galactic Plane from UHURU. *Astrophys. J.*, 165:L27.

[Gilman et al., 1986] Gilman, D. A., Hurley, K. C., Seward, F. D., Schnopper, H. W., Sullivan, J. D., and Metzger, A. E. (1986). An Upper Limit to X-Ray Emission from Saturn. *Astrophys. J.*, 300:453.

[Girardi et al., 1996] Girardi, M., Fadda, D., Giuricin, G., Mardirossian, F., Mezzetti, M., and Biviano, A. (1996). Velocity Dispersions and X-Ray Temperatures of Galaxy Clusters. *Astrophys. J.*, 457:61.

[gM.A., 1910] gM.A., S. C. (1910). Xxxvi. the sine condition in relation to the coma of optical systems. *The London, Edinburgh, and Dublin Philosophical Magazine and Journal of Science*, 19(111):356–365.

[Gondoin et al., 2000] Gondoin, P., Aschenbach, B., Erd, C., Lumb, D. H., Majerowicz, S., Neumann, D., and Sauvageot, J. L. (2000). In-orbit calibration of the XMM-Newton telescopes. In Flanagan, K. A. and Siegmund, O. H., editors, *X-Ray and Gamma-Ray Instrumentation for Astronomy XI*, volume 4140 of *Society of Photo-Optical Instrumentation Engineers (SPIE) Conference Series*, pages 1–12.

[Gorenstein et al., 1970] Gorenstein, P., Kellogg, E. M., and Gursky, H. (1970). X-Ray Characteristics of Three Supernova Remnants. *Astrophys. J.*, 160:199.

[Greene, 2017] Greene, J. E. (2017). Review article: Tracing the recorded history of thin-film sputter deposition: From the 1800s to 2017. *Journal of Vacuum Science & Technology A*, 35(5):05C204.

[Grimmer et al., 2001] Grimmer, H., Zaharko, O., Mertins, H. C., and Schäfers, F. (2001). Polarizing mirrors for soft X-ray radiation. *Nuclear Instruments and Methods in Physics Research A*, 467:354–357.

[Gruber et al., 1996] Gruber, D. E., Blanco, P. R., Heindl, W. A., Pelling, M. R., Rothschild, R. E., and Hink, P. L. (1996). The high energy X-ray timing experiment on XTE. *Astron. Astrophys. Suppl.*, 120:641–644.

[Güdel et al., 2001] Güdel, M., Audard, M., Briggs, K., Haberl, F., Magee, H., Maggio, A., Mewe, R., Pallavicini, R., and Pye, J. (2001). The XMM-Newton view of stellar coronae: X-ray spectroscopy of the corona of ¡ASTROBJ¿AB Doradus¡/ASTROBJ¿. *Astron. Astrophys.*, 365:L336–L343.

[Gutman, 1994] Gutman, G. (1994). High-performance mo/si and w/b4c multilayer mirrors for soft x-ray imaging optics. *J Xray Sci Technology*, 4.

[Harrison and NuSTAR Science Team, 2004] Harrison, F. and NuSTAR Science Team (2004). Nuclear Spectroscopic Telescope Array (NuSTAR) mission: Imaging the Hard X-ray Sky. In *AAS/High Energy Astrophysics Division #8*, AAS/High Energy Astrophysics Division, page 41.05.

[Heilmann et al., 2009] Heilmann, R. K., Ahn, M., Flanagan, K. A., Huenemoerder, D. P., and Schattenburg, M. L. (2009). Soft X-Ray Critical-Angle Transmission Grating Spectrometer for the International X-Ray Observatory. In *American Astronomical Society Meeting Abstracts #213*, volume 213 of *American Astronomical Society Meeting Abstracts*, page 457.10.

[Heitler, 1954] Heitler, W. (1954). *Quantum theory of radiation.*

[Hermsen and Winkler, 1998] Hermsen, W. and Winkler, C. (1998). The INTEGRAL Mission. In Koyama, K., Kitamoto, S., and Itoh, M., editors, *The Hot Universe*, volume 188 of *IAU Symposium*, page 87.

[Hill et al., 1999] Hill, J. E., Burrows, D. N., Nousek, J. A., Wells, A., Turner, M., Willingale, R., Holland, A., Citterio, O., Chincarini, G., Campana, S., Tagliaferri, G., and Swift XRT Team (1999). The Swift X-ray Telescope. In *American Astronomical Society Meeting Abstracts*, volume 195, page 71.01.

[Hong et al., 2014] Hong, J., Grindlay, J., Romaine, S., Ramsey, B., Binzel, R. P., Boynton, W., Georenstein, P., Kraft, R., Kenter, A., Elvis, M., Wolk, S., Smith, R., Lim, L., Lisse, C., Branduardi- Raymont, G., Allen, B., and Lee, J. (2014).

Miniature Lightweight X-Ray Optics (MiXO) for Solar System Exploration. In *Lunar and Planetary Science Conference*, page 2203.

[Hull, 1921] Hull, A. W. (1921). The effect of a uniform magnetic field on the motion of electrons between coaxial cylinders. *Phys. Rev.*, 18:31–57.

[Hundhausen, 1968] Hundhausen, A. J. (1968). Direct Observations of Solar-Wind Particles. *Space Sci. Rev.*, 8:690–749.

[Ilovaisky and Ryter, 1972] Ilovaisky, S. A. and Ryter, C. (1972). Soft X-Rays from Supernova Remnants. *Astron. Astrophys.*, 18:163.

[Jach et al., 2009] Jach, T., Ullom, J. N., and Elam, W. T. (2009). The microcalorimeter X-ray detector: A true paradigm shift in X-ray spectroscopy. *European Physical Journal Special Topics*, 169:237–242.

[Jagoda et al., 1972] Jagoda, N., Austin, G., Mickiewicz, S., and Goddard, R. (1972). The UHURU X-Ray Instrument. *IEEE Transactions on Nuclear Science*, 19:579.

[Jankowski and Makowiecki, 1991] Jankowski, A. F. and Makowiecki, D. M. (1991). W/b4c multilayer x-ray mirrors. *Optical Engineering*, 30:30 – 30 – 7.

[Jankowski. et al., 1990] Jankowski., A. F., Schrawyer, L. R., and Wall, M. A. (1990). Structural stability of heattreated w/c and w/b4c multilayers. *Journal of Applied Physics*, 68(10):5162–5168.

[Jankowski et al., 1989] Jankowski, A. F., Schrawyer, L. R., Wall, M. A., Craig, W. W., Morales, R. I., and Makowieck, D. M. (1989). Interfacial bonding in w/c and w/b4c multilayers. *Journal of Vacuum Science & Technology A*, 7(4):2914–2918.

[Jiang et al., 2015] Jiang, H., Yan, S., Zhu, J., Dong, Z., Zheng, Y., He, Y., and Li, A. (2015). Investigation of defects in sputtered w/b4c multilayers. *Applied Surface Science*, 357:1180 – 1186.

[Jones et al., 1979] Jones, C., Mandel, E., Schwarz, J., Forman, W., Murray, S. S., and Harnden, F. R., J. (1979). The structure and evolution of X-ray clusters. *Astrophys. J.*, 234:L21–L25.

[Kallio et al., 1997] Kallio, E., Luhmann, J. G., and Barabash, S. (1997). Charge exchange near mars: The solar wind absorption and energetic neutral atom production. *Journal of Geophysical Research: Space Physics*, 102(A10):22183–22197.

[Kislat et al., 2015] Kislat, F., Clark, B., Beilicke, M., and Krawczynski, H. (2015). Analyzing the data from X-ray polarimeters with Stokes parameters. *Astroparticle Physics*, 68:45–51.

[Koch-Miramond, 1985] Koch-Miramond, L. (1985). *XMM: The X-ray Multiple Mirror Observatory*, page 291.

[Krasnopolsky et al., 2004] Krasnopolsky, V. A., Greenwood, J. B., and Stancil, P. C. (2004). X-Ray and extreme ultraviolet emissions from comets. *Space Sci. Rev.*, 113:271–374.

[Krawczynski et al., 2011] Krawczynski, H., Garson, A., Guo, Q., Baring, M. G., Ghosh, P., Beilicke, M., and Lee, K. (2011). Scientific prospects for hard X-ray polarimetry. *Astroparticle Physics*, 34:550–567.

[Krawczynski et al., 2016] Krawczynski, H. S., Stern, D., Harrison, F. A., Kislat, F. F., Zajczyk, A., Beilicke, M., Hoormann, J., Guo, Q., Endsley, R., Ingram, A. R., Miyasaka, H., Madsen, K. K., Aaron, K. M., Amini, R., Baring, M. G., Beheshtipour, B., Bodaghee, A., Booth, J., Borden, C., Böttcher,

M., Christensen, F. E., Coppi, P. S., Cowsik, R., Davis, S., Dexter, J., Done, C., Dominguez, L. A., Ellison, D., English, R. J., Fabian, A. C., Falcone, A., Favretto, J. A., Fernández, R., Giommi, P., Grefenstette, B. W., Kara, E., Lee, C. H., Lyutikov, M., Maccarone, T., Matsumoto, H., McKinney, J., Mihara, T., Miller, J. M., Narayan, R., Natalucci, L., Özel, F., Pivovaroff, M. J., Pravdo, S., Psaltis, D., Okajima, T., Toma, K., and Zhang, W. W. (2016). X-ray polarimetry with the Polarization Spectroscopic Telescope Array (PolSTAR). *Astroparticle Physics*, 75:8–28.

[Krieger et al., 1997] Krieger, A. S., Parsignault, D., Ulmer, M. P., and Altkorn, R. A. (1997). Focusing X-ray Optics for 40-100 keV. In *American Astronomical Society Meeting Abstracts #190*, volume 190 of *American Astronomical Society Meeting Abstracts*, page 10.05.

[Kundu, 1961] Kundu, M. R. (1961). Bursts of Centimeter-Wave Emission and the Region of Origin of X Rays from Solar Flares. *Journal of Geophysical Research*, 66:4308–4312.

[Kunieda et al., 2006] Kunieda, H., Mitsuda, K., Takahashi, T., Kelley, R., and White, N. (2006). Current status of Suzaku and its early results. In *Society of Photo-Optical Instrumentation Engineers (SPIE) Conference Series*, volume 6266, page 626605.

[Liang, 1979] Liang, E. P. T. (1979). On the hard X-ray emission mechanism of active galactic nuclei sources. *Astrophys. J. Lett.*, 231:L111–L114.

[Lisse, 2001] Lisse, C. M. (2001). Observational Trends of Cometary X-ray Emission. In *AGU Spring Meeting Abstracts*, volume 2001, pages SH21A–03 INVITED.

[Lisse et al., 1999] Lisse, C. M., Christian, D., Dennerl, K., Englhauser, J., Trümper, J., Desch, M., Marshall, F. E., Petre, R., and Snowden, S. (1999). X-Ray and Extreme Ultraviolet Emission from Comet P/Encke 1997. *Icarus*, 141:316–330.

[Lisse et al., 2004] Lisse, C. M., Cravens, T. E., and Dennerl, K. (2004). *X-ray and extreme ultraviolet emission from comets*, page 631.

[Lisse et al., 1996] Lisse, C. M., Dennerl, K., Englhauser, J., Harden, M., Marshall, F. E., Mumma, M. J., Petre, R., Pye, J. P., Ricketts, M. J., Schmitt, J., Trumper, J., and West, R. G. (1996). Discovery of X-ray and Extreme Ultraviolet Emission from Comet C/Hyakutake 1996 B2. *Science*, 274:205–209.

[Lotti et al., 2014] Lotti, S., Cea, D., Macculi, C., Mineo, T., Natalucci, L., Perinati, E., Piro, L., Federici, M., and Martino, B. (2014). In-orbit background of X-ray microcalorimeters and its effects on observations. *Astron. Astrophys.*, 569:A54.

[MacFadyen and Woosley, 1999] MacFadyen, A. I. and Woosley, S. E. (1999). Collapsars: Gamma-Ray Bursts and Explosions in "Failed Supernovae". *Astrophys. J.*, 524:262–289.

[Maeda et al., 2015] Maeda, Y., Ichihara, K., Kan, H., Shionome, Y., Sato, T., Sato, T., Hayashi, T., Ishida, M., Namba, Y., Takahashi, H., Miyazawa, T., Ishibashi, K., Sakai, M., Sugita, S., Haba, Y., Matsumoto, H., and Mori, H. (2015). Thermal stress test of the depth-graded platinum/carbon reflectors. *Journal of Astronomical Telescopes and Instruments and and Systems*, 1:1 – 1 – 4.

[Majhi et al., 2018] Majhi, A., Dilliwar, M., Pradhan, P. C., Jena, S., Nayak, M., Singh, M. N., Udupa, D. V., and Sahoo, N. K. (2018). Evaluation of microstructure and residual stress in w/b4c multilayer optics. *Journal of Applied Physics*, 124(11):115306.

[Mandel'Shtam et al., 1968] Mandel'Shtam, S. L., Tindo, I. P., Cheremukhin, G. S., Sorokin, L. S., and Dmitriev, A. B. (1968). Lunar X Rays and the Cosmic X-Ray Background Measured by the Lunar Satellite Luna-12. *Cosmic Research*, 6:100–106.

[Mao et al., 1997] Mao, P. H., Harrison, F. A., Platonov, Y. Y., Broadway, D., Degroot, B., Christensen, F. E., Craig, W. W., and Hailey, C. J. (1997). Development of grazing incidence multilayer mirrors for hard x-ray focusing telescopes. In Siegmund, O. H. and Gummin, M. A., editors, *EUV, X-Ray, and Gamma-Ray Instrumentation for Astronomy VIII*, volume 3114 of *Society of Photo-Optical Instrumentation Engineers (SPIE) Conference Series*, pages 526–534.

[Marar et al., 1981] Marar, T. M. K., Sharma, D. P., Kasturirangan, K., and Rao, U. R. (1981). On the origin of the gamma ray burst of March 5, 1979. *International Cosmic Ray Conference*, 9:44–47.

[Marshall, 2015] Marshall, H. (2015). Rocket Experiment Demonstration of a Soft X-ray Polarimeter. NASA APRA Proposal.

[Marshall et al., 2010] Marshall, H. L., Heilmann, R. K., Schulz, N. S., and Murphy, K. D. (2010). Broadband soft x-ray polarimetry. In *Space Telescopes and Instrumentation 2010: Ultraviolet to Gamma Ray*, volume 7732 of *Society of Photo-Optical Instrumentation Engineers (SPIE) Conference Series*, page 77320F.

[Marshall et al., 1998] Marshall, H. L., Murray, S. S., Silver, E., Schnopper, H., and Weisskopf, M. C. (1998). A Polarimeter for Low Energy X-ray Astrophysical

Sources (PLEXAS). In *American Astronomical Society Meeting Abstracts #192*, volume 192 of *American Astronomical Society Meeting Abstracts*, page 35.04.

[Marshall et al., 2014] Marshall, H. L., Schulz, N. S., Windt, D. L., Gullikson, E. M., Blake, E., Getty, D., and McInturff, Z. (2014). The use of laterally graded multilayer mirrors for soft X-ray polarimetry. In *Space Telescopes and Instrumentation 2014: Ultraviolet to Gamma Ray*, volume 9144 of *Society of Photo-Optical Instrumentation Engineers (SPIE) Conference Series*, page 91441K.

[Matteson, 1974] Matteson, J. L. (1974). The HEAO-A Satellite and its Capabilities to Study the Cosmic Gamma-Ray Bursts. In Strong, I. B., editor, *Transient Cosmic Gamma- and X-Ray Sources*, page 237.

[Maurellis and Cravens, 2001] Maurellis, A. N. and Cravens, T. E. (2001). X-Ray Emission From Planetary Atmospheres due to the Scattering and Fluorescence of Solar Photons. In *AGU Spring Meeting Abstracts*, volume 2001, pages SH21A-10.

[Meltzer and Thorne, 1966] Meltzer, D. W. and Thorne, K. S. (1966). Normal Modes of Radial Pulsation of Stars at the End Point of Thermonuclear Evolution. *Astrophys. J.*, 145:514.

[Metzger et al., 1980] Metzger, A. E., Gilman, D. A., Luthey, J. L., Hurley, K. C., Sullivan, J. D., Seward, F. D., and Schnopper, H. W. (1980). Observation of X-Rays from the Jovian System. In *Bulletin of the American Astronomical Society*, volume 12, page 450.

[Metzger et al., 1983] Metzger, A. E., Luthey, J. L., Gilman, D. A., Hurley, K. C., Schnopper, H. W., Seward, F. D., and Sullivan, J. D. (1983). The detection of X rays from Jupiter. *J. Geophys. Res.*, 88:7731-7741.

[Michel, 1964] Michel, F. C. (1964). Interaction between the solar wind and the lunar atmosphere. *Planetary and Space Science*, 12:1075–1091.

[Michette, 1986] Michette, A. G. (1986). *Optical systems for soft X rays*. New York : Plenum Press. Includes index.

[Modi et al., 2019] Modi, M. H., Gupta, R. K., Kane, S. R., Prasad, V., Garg, C. K., Yadav, P., Raghuvanshi, V. K., Singh, A., and Sinha, M. (2019). A soft x-ray reflectivity beamline for 100-1500 ev energy range at indus-2 synchrotron radiation source. *AIP Conference Proceedings*, 2054(1):060022.

[Moseley et al., 1985] Moseley, S. H., Kelley, R. L., Mather, J. C., Mushotzky, R. F., Szymkowiak, A. E., and McCammon, D. (1985). Thermal detectors as single photon X-ray spectrometers. *IEEE Transactions on Nuclear Science*, 32:134–138.

[Mumma et al., 1997] Mumma, M. J., Krasnopolsky, V. A., and Abbott, M. J. (1997). Soft X-Rays From Four Comets Observed With EUVE. *Astrophys. J.*, 491:L125–L128.

[Mushotzky et al., 1993] Mushotzky, R. F., Done, C., and Pounds, K. A. (1993). X-ray spectra and time variability of active galactic nuclei. *Annual Review of Astronomy and Astrophysics*, 31:717–717.

[Nandra et al., 1991] Nandra, K., Pounds, K. A., Stewart, G. C., George, I. M., Hayashida, K., Makino, F., and Ohashi, T. (1991). Compton reflection and the variable X-ray spectrum of NGC 5548. *Mon. Not. Roy. Astron. Soc.*, 248:760.

[Narendranath et al., 2010] Narendranath, K. C. S., Athiray, P. S., Unnikrishann, U., Sreekumar, P., C1XS Team Grande, M., Cook, A., Wilding, M., Carter,

J. A., Maddison, B. J., Kellett, B. J., Howe, C. J., Swinyard, B. M., Sreeku-
mar, P., Shrivastava, A., Narendranath, S., Huovelin, J., Alha, L., Crawford,
I., Joy, K. H., Weider, S. Z., Duston, C. L., Gasnaut, O., Maurice, S., Smith,
D., Rothery, D., Anand, M., Holland, A., Gow, J., Russell, S., Goswami, J. N.,
Bhandari, N., Lawrence, D., Fernandes, V., Okada, T., Koschny, D., Pieters,
C., and Wieczorek, M. (2010). Analysis of Lunar X-Ray Data: Line Flux to
Elemental Abundance from the C1XS Experiment on Chandrayaan-1. In *Work-
shop X-ray Fluorescence Spectroscopy in Planetary Remote Sensing*, volume 687
of *ESA Special Publication*, page 6.

[Narendranath et al., 2011] Narendranath, S., Athiray, P. S., Sreekumar, P., Kellett, B. J., Alha, L., Howe, C. J., Joy, K. H., Grande, M., Huovelin, J., Crawford,
I. A., Unnikrishnan, U., Lalita, S., Subramaniam, S., Weider, S. Z., Nittler,
L. R., Gasnault, O., Rothery, D., Fernandes, V. A., Bhandari, N., Goswami,
J. N., Wieczorek, M. A., and the C1XS Team (2011). Lunar X-ray fluorescence
observations by the Chandrayaan-1 X-ray Spectrometer (C1XS): Results from
the nearside southern highlands. *Icarus*, 214:53–66.

[Nayak et al., 2012] Nayak, M., N. Rao, P., and Lodha, G. (2012). Magnetron
sputtering system for fabrication of x-ray multilayer optics. *Asian J. Physics*.

[Nigam, 1965] Nigam, A. N. (1965). Origin of Anomalous Surface Reflection of X
Rays. *Physical Review*, 138:1189–1191.

[Oda et al., 1976] Oda, M., Muranaka, N., Matsuoka, M., Miyamoto, S., and
Ogawara, Y. (1976). The Design and Construction of Modulation Collimators.
Space Science Instrumentation, 2:141.

[Okada et al., 1994] Okada, H., Mayama, K., Goto, Y., Kusunoki, I., and Yanagihara, M. (1994). Thermal stability of sputtered mo/x and w/x (x = bn:o, b4c:o, si, and c) multiplayer soft-x-ray mirrors. *Appl. Opt.*, 33(19):4219–4224.

[Panini et al., 2018] Panini, S. S., Nayak, M., Narendranath, K. C. S., Pradhan, P. C., Athiray, P., Sreekumar, P., Lodha, G., and Tiwari, M. K. (2018). Development of multilayer mirrors for space-based astronomical x-ray optics. *Journal of Optics*, 47(1):91–95.

[Panini et al., 2018] Panini, S. S., Sreekumar, P., Marshall, H. L., Narendranath, S., Nayak, M., and Athiray, P. S. (2018). Multilayer mirror-based soft x-ray polarimeter for astronomical observations. *Journal of Astronomical Telescopes, Instruments, and Systems*, 4:011002.

[Payne, 1979] Payne, D. G. (1979). *X-Rays from Active Galactic Nuclei: Emission Mechanisms and Interaction with Ambient Media*. PhD thesis, Yale University., New Haven, CT.

[Peterson, 1975] Peterson, L. E. (1975). Instrumental technique in X-ray astronomy. *Annual Review of Astronomy and Astrophysics*, 13:423–509.

[Petrosian et al., 1979] Petrosian, V., Langer, S. H., and Frost, K. J. (1979). The Scattering of Solar Flare X-Rays in the Earth's Atmosphere. In *Bulletin of the American Astronomical Society*, volume 11, page 440.

[Pradhan et al., 2018] Pradhan, P. C., Majhi, A., and Nayak, M. (2018). Optical performance of w/b4c multilayer mirror in the soft x-ray region. *Journal of Applied Physics*, 123(9):095302.

[Predehl et al., 2007] Predehl, P., Andritschke, R., Bornemann, W., Bräuninger, H., Briel, U., Brunner, H., Burkert, W., Dennerl, K., Eder, J., Freyberg, M.,

Friedrich, P., Fürmetz, M., Hartmann, R., Hartner, G., Hasinger, G., Herrmann, S., Holl, P., Huber, H., Kendziorra, E., Kink, W., Meidinger, N., Müller, S., Pavlinsky, M., Pfeffermann, E., Rohé, C., Santangelo, A., Schmitt, J., Schwope, A., Steinmetz, M., Strüder, L., Sunyaev, R., Tiedemann, L., Vongehr, M., Wilms, J., Erhard, M., Gutruf, S., Jugler, D., Kampf, D., Graue, R., Citterio, O., Valsecci, G., Vernani, D., and Zimmerman, M. (2007). eROSITA. In *UV, X-Ray, and Gamma-Ray Space Instrumentation for Astronomy XV*, volume 6686 of *Society of Photo-Optical Instrumentation Engineers (SPIE) Conference Series*, page 668617.

[Rao et al., 2013] Rao, P. N., Rai, S. K., Nayak, M., and Lodha, G. S. (2013). Stability and normal incidence reflectivity of w/b4c multilayer mirror near the boron k absorption edge. *Appl. Opt.*, 52(25):6126–6130.

[Reeves et al., 2002] Reeves, J. N., Watson, D., Osborne, J. P., Pounds, K. A., O'Brien, P. T., Short, A. D. T., Turner, M. J. L., Watson, M. G., Mason, K. O., Ehle, M., and Schartel, N. (2002). The signature of supernova ejecta in the X-ray afterglow of the γ-ray burst 011211. *Nature*, 416:512–515.

[Rntgen, 1896] Rntgen, W. C. (1896). On a new kind of rays. *Science*, 3(59):227–231.

[Romani, 1996] Romani, R. W. (1996). Gamma-Ray Pulsars: Radiation Processes in the Outer Magnetosphere. *Astrophys. J.*, 470:469.

[Romani and Watters, 2010] Romani, R. W. and Watters, K. P. (2010). Constraining Pulsar Magnetosphere Geometry with γ-ray Light Curves. *Astrophys. J.*, 714:810–824.

[Rosen. et al., 2016] Rosen., S. R., Webb, N. A., Watson, M. G., Ballet, J., Barret, D., Braito, V., Carrera, F. J., Ceballos, M. T., Coriat, M., Ceca, R. D., Denkinson, G., Esquej, P., Farrell, S. A., Freyberg, M., Grisé, F., Guillout, P., Heil, L., Koliopanos, F., Law-Green, D., Lamer, G., Lin, D., Martino, R., Michel, L., Motch, C., Gomez-Moran, A. N., Page, C. G., Page, K., Page, M., Pakull, M. W., Pye, J., Read, A., Rodriguez, P., Sakano, M., Saxton, R., Schwope, A., Scott, A. E., Sturm, R., Traulsen, I., Yershov, V., and Zolotukhin, I. (2016). The xmm-newton serendipitous survey. vii. the third xmm-newton serendipitous source catalogue. *Astron. Astrophys.*, 590:A1.

[Rosner et al., 1985] Rosner, R., Golub, L., and Vaiana, G. S. (1985). On stellar x-ray emission. *Annual Review of Astronomy and Astrophysics*, 23(1):413–452.

[Rosner and Vaiana, 1980] Rosner, R. and Vaiana, G. S. (1980). Stellar Coronae from Einstein: Observations and Theory. In Giacconi, R. and Setti, G., editors, *NATO Advanced Science Institutes (ASI) Series C*, volume 60, page 129.

[Roy et al., 1977] Roy, A., Ballas, J., Jagoda, N., McKinnon, P., Ramsey, A., and Wester, E. (1977). The HEAO-A scanning modulation collimator instrument. *IEEE Transactions on Nuclear Science*, 24:804–809.

[Scarsi, 1997] Scarsi, L. (1997). The BeppoSAX mission. In *Data Analysis in Astronomy*, pages 65–78.

[Schatzman, 1949] Schatzman, E. (1949). The heating of the solar corona and chromosphere. *Annales d'Astrophysique*, 12:203.

[Schmitt et al., 1991] Schmitt, J. H. M. M., Snowden, S. L., Aschenbach, B., Hasinger, G., Pfeffermann, E., Predehl, P., and Trumper, J. (1991). A soft X-ray image of the Moon. *Nature*, 349:583–587.

[Schnittman and Krolik, 2009] Schnittman, J. D. and Krolik, J. H. (2009). X-ray Polarization from Accreting Black Holes: The Thermal State. *Astrophys. J.*, 701:1175–1187.

[Schnittman and Krolik, 2010] Schnittman, J. D. and Krolik, J. H. (2010). X-ray Polarization from Accreting Black Holes: Coronal Emission. *Astrophys. J.*, 712:908–924.

[Schonherr, G. and Wilms, J. and Kretschmar, P. and Kreykenbohm, I. and Santangelo, A. and Ro Schonherr, G. and Wilms, J. and Kretschmar, P. and Kreykenbohm, I. and Santangelo, A. and Rothschild, R. E. and Coburn, W. and Staubert, R., title = "A model for cyclotron resonance scattering features", j. . *Astron. Astrophys.*. k. . X. y. . . m. . S. v. . . p. . . d. . . a. . a. e. . . p. . a. a. . h. a. . P.

[Schwartz et al., 1972] Schwartz, D. A., Boldt, E. A., Holt, S. S., Serlemitsos, P. J., and Bleach, R. D. (1972). A high sensitivity search for X-rays from supernova remnants in Aquila. In *Bulletin of the American Astronomical Society*, volume 4, page 261.

[Seetha et al., 2006] Seetha, S., Ramadevi, M. C., Babu, V. C., Sharma, M. R., Murthy, N. S. R., Ashoka, B. N., Shyama, K. C., Kulkarni, R., Meena, G., and Sreekumar, P. (2006). The Scanning Sky Monitor (SSM) on ASTROSAT. *Advances in Space Research*, 38:2995–2998.

[Seward et al., 1976] Seward, F. D., Horton, B., Pollard, G., and Sanford, P. W. (1976). Argon fluorescent X rays in the Earth's atmosphere during solar flares. *Nature*, 264:421–423.

[Shamu, 1961] Shamu, R. E. (1961). High-pressure gas scintillation counters. *Nuclear Instruments and Methods*, 14:297–301.

[She et al., 2015] She, R., Feng, H., Muleri, F., Soffitta, P., Xu, R., Li, H., Bellazzini, R., Wang, Z., Spiga, D., Minuti, M., Brez, A., Spandre, G., Pinchera, M., Sgrò, C., Baldini, L., Wen, M., Shen, Z., Pareschi, G., Tagliaferri, G., Tayabaly, K., Salmaso, B., and Zhan, Y. (2015). LAMP: a micro-satellite based soft x-ray polarimeter for astrophysics. In *UV, X-Ray, and Gamma-Ray Space Instrumentation for Astronomy XIX*, volume 9601 of *Society of Photo-Optical Instrumentation Engineers (SPIE) Conference Series*, page 96010I.

[Singam et al., 2018] Singam, P. S., Nayak, M., Gupta, R., Pradhan, P. C., and Shyama Narendranath, A. M., and Sreekumar, P. (2018). Thermal and temporal stability of ¡italic¿w¡/italic¿¡inline-formula¿ ¡mml:math display="inline" xmlns:mml="http://www.w3.org/1998/math/mathml"¿ ¡mml:mrow¿ ¡mml:mo stretchy="false"¿/¡/mml:mo¿ ¡/mml:mrow¿ ¡/mml:math¿ ¡/inline-formula¿¡italic¿b¡/italic¿¡sub¿4¡/sub¿¡italic¿c¡/italic¿ multilayer mirrors for space-based astronomical applications. *Journal of Astronomical Telescopes, Instruments, and Systems*, 4:4 − 4 − 8.

[Singh et al., 2017a] Singh, K. P., Stewart, G. C., Westergaard, N. J., Bhattacharayya, S., Chandra, S., Chitnis, V. R., Dewangan, G. C., Kothare, A. T., Mirza, I. M., Mukerjee, K., Navalkar, V., Shah, H., Abbey, A. F., Beardmore, A. P., Kotak, S., Kamble, N., Vishwakarama, S., Pathare, D. P., Risbud, V. M., Koyande, J. P., Stevenson, T., Bicknell, C., Crawford, T., Hansford, G., Peters, G., Sykes, J., Agarwal, P., Sebastian, M., Rajarajan, A., Nagesh, G., Narendra, S., Ramesh, M., Rai, R., Navalgund, K. H., Sarma, K. S., Pandiyan, R., Subbarao, K., Gupta, T., Thakkar, N., Singh, A. K., and Bajpai, A. (2017a). Soft X-ray Focusing Telescope Aboard AstroSat: Design, Characteristics and Performance. *Journal of Astrophysics and Astronomy*, 38:29.

[Singh et al., 2017b] Singh, K. P., Stewart, G. C., Westergaard, N. J., Bhattacharayya, S., Chandra, S., Chitnis, V. R., Dewangan, G. C., Kothare, A. T., Mirza, I. M., Mukerjee, K., Navalkar, V., Shah, H., Abbey, A. F., Beardmore, A. P., Kotak, S., Kamble, N., Vishwakarama, S., Pathare, D. P., Risbud, V. M., Koyande, J. P., Stevenson, T., Bicknell, C., Crawford, T., Hansford, G., Peters,

G., Sykes, J., Agarwal, P., Sebastian, M., Rajarajan, A., Nagesh, G., Narendra, S., Ramesh, M., Rai, R., Navalgund, K. H., Sarma, K. S., Pandiyan, R., Subbarao, K., Gupta, T., Thakkar, N., Singh, A. K., and Bajpai, A. (2017b). Soft X-ray Focusing Telescope Aboard AstroSat: Design, Characteristics and Performance. *Journal of Astrophysics and Astronomy*, 38:29.

[Soltau et al., 1996] Soltau, H., Holl, P., Kemmer, J., Krisch, S., Zanthier, C. V., Hauff, D., Richter, R., Bräuninger, H., Hartmann, R., Hartner, G., Krause, N., Meidinger, N., Pfeffermann, E., Reppin, C., Schwaab, G., Strüder, L., Trümper, J., Kendziorra, E., and Krämer, J. (1996). Performance of the pn-CCD X-ray detector system designed for the XMM satellite mission. *Nuclear Instruments and Methods in Physics Research A*, 377A:340–345.

[Spiller, 1996] Spiller, E. (1996). Soft X-Ray Optics. *Optics & Photonics News*, 7:60.

[Spreiter and Alksne, 1970] Spreiter, J. R. and Alksne, A. Y. (1970). Solar-wind flow past objects in the solar system. *Annual Review of Fluid Mechanics*, 2:313–354.

[Stokes, 1851] Stokes, G. G. (1851). On the Composition and Resolution of Streams of Polarized Light from different Sources. *Transactions of the Cambridge Philosophical Society*, 9:399.

[Stoney, 1918] Stoney, G. (1918). Stresses in turbine blading. *Journal of the American Society for Naval Engineers*, 30(3):599–606.

[Sun and Richardson, 1954] Sun, C. R. and Richardson, J. R. (1954). A Multiple-Wire Proportional Counter for Fast Neutron Detection. *Review of Scientific Instruments*, 25:691–694.

[Sunyaev and Titarchuk, 1985] Sunyaev, R. A. and Titarchuk, L. G. (1985). Comptonization of low-frequency radiation in accretion disks Angular distribution and polarization of hard radiation. *Astron. Astrophys.*, 143:374–388.

[Takahara et al., 1981] Takahara, F., Tsuruta, S., and Ichimaru, S. (1981). X-rays from active galactic nuclei. *Astrophys. J.*, 251:26–30.

[Takahashi et al., 2018] Takahashi, T., Kokubun, M., Mitsuda, K., Kelley, R. L., Ohashi, T., Aharonian, F., Akamatsu, H., Akimoto, F., Allen, S. W., Anabuki, N., Angelini, L., Arnaud, K., Asai, M., Audard, M., Awaki, H., Axelsson, M., Azzarello, P., Baluta, C., Bamba, A., Bando, N., Bautz, M. W., Bialas, T., Blandford, R., Boyce, K., Brenneman, L. W., Brown, G. V., Bulbul, E., Cackett, E. M., Canavan, E., Chernyakova, M., Chiao, M. P., Coppi, P. S., Costantini, E., O'Dell, S., DiPirro, M., Done, C., Dotani, T., Doty, J., Ebisawa, K., Eckart, M. E., Enoto, T., Ezoe, Y., Fabian, A. C., Ferrigno, C., Foster, A. R., Fujimoto, R., Fukazawa, Y., Funk, S., Furuzawa, A., Galeazzi, M., Gallo, L. C., Gandhi, P., Gilmore, K., Giustini, M., Goldwurm, A., Gu, L., Guainazzi, M., Haas, D., Haba, Y., Hagino, K., Hamaguchi, K., Harrus, I. M., Hatsukade, I., Hayashi, T., Hayashi, K., Hayashida, K., den Herder, J.-W., Hiraga, J. S., Hirose, K., Hornschemeier, A., Hoshino, A., Hughes, J. P., Ichinohe, Y., Iizuka, R., Inoue, H., Inoue, Y., Ishibashi, K., Ishida, M., Ishikawa, K., Ishimura, K., Ishisaki, Y., Itoh, M., Iwai, M., Iwata, N., Iyomoto, N., Jewell, C., Kaastra, J., Kallman, T., Kamae, T., Kara, E., Kataoka, J., Katsuda, S., Katsuta, J., Kawaharada, M., Kawai, N., Kawano, T., Kawasaki, S., Khangulyan, D., Kilbourne, C. A., Kimball, M., King, A., Kitaguchi, T., Kitamoto, S., Kitayama, T., Kohmura, T., Konami, S., Kosaka, T., Koujelev, A., Koyama, K., Koyama, S., Kretschmar, P., Krimm, H. A., Kubota, A., Kunieda, H., Laurent, P., Lee, S.-H., Leutenegger, M. A., Limousin, O., Loewenstein, M., Long, K. S., Lumb,

D., Madejski, G., Maeda, Y., Maier, D., Makishima, K., Markevitch, M., Masters, C., Matsumoto, H., Matsushita, K., McCammon, D., Mcguinness, D., McNamara, B. R., Mehdipour, M., Miko, J., Miller, E. D., Miller, J. M., Mineshige, S., Minesugi, K., Mitsuishi, I., Miyazawa, T., Mizuno, T., Mori, H., Mori, K., Moroso, F., Moseley, H., Muench, T., Mukai, K., Murakami, H., Murakami, T., Mushotzky, R. F., Nagano, H., Nagino, R., Nakagawa, T., Nakajima, H., Nakamori, T., Nakano, T., Nakashima, S., Nakazawa, K., Namba, Y., Natsukari, C., Nishioka, Y., Nobukawa, K. K., Nobukawa, M., Noda, H., Nomachi, M., Odaka, H., Ogawa, H., Ogawa, M., Ogi, K., Ohno, M., Ohta, M., Okajima, T., Okamoto, A., Okazaki, T., Ota, N., Ozaki, M., Paerels, F., Paltani, S., Parmar, A., Petre, R., Pinto, C., de Plaa, J., Pohl, M., Pontius, J., Porter, F. S., Pottschmidt, K., Ramsey, B., Reynolds, C., Russell, H., Safi-Harb, S., Saito, S., Sakai, K., Sakai, S.-i., Sameshima, H., Sasaki, T., Sato, G., Sato, K., Sato, R., Sato, Y., Sawada, M., Schartel, N., Serlemitsos, P. J., Seta, H., Shibano, Y., Shida, M., Shidatsu, M., Shimada, T., Shinozaki, K., Shirron, P., Simionescu, A., Simmons, C., Smith, R. K., Sneiderman, G., Soong, Y., Stawarz, Ł., Sugawara, Y., Sugita, S., Sugita, H., Szymkowiak, A., Tajima, H., Takahashi, H., Takeda, S., Takei, Y., Tamagawa, T., Tamura, T., Tamura, K., Tanaka, T., Tanaka, Y., Tanaka, Y. T., Tashiro, M. S., Tawara, Y., Terada, Y., Terashima, Y., Tombesi, F., Tomida, H., Tsuboi, Y., Tsujimoto, M., Tsunemi, H., Tsuru, T. G., Uchida, H., Uchiyama, H., Uchiyama, Y., Ueda, S., Ueda, Y., Ueno, S., Uno, S., Urry, C. M., Ursino, E., de Vries, C. P., Wada, A., Watanabe, S., Watanabe, T., Werner, N., Wik, D. R., Wilkins, D. R., Williams, B. J., Yamada, S., Yamada, T., Yamaguchi, H., Yamaoka, K., Yamasaki, N. Y., Yamauchi, M., Yamauchi, S., Yaqoob, T., Yatsu, Y., Yonetoku, D., Yoshida, A., Yuasa, T., Zhuravleva, I., and Zoghbi, A. (2018). Hitomi (ASTRO-H) X-ray Astronomy Satellite. *Journal of Astronomical Telescopes, Instruments, and*

Systems, 4:021402.

[Tawara et al., 1998] Tawara, Y., Yamashita, K., Kunieda, H., Tamura, K., Furuzawa, A., Haga, K., Nakajo, N., Okajima, T., Takata, H., Serlemitsos, P. J., Tueller, J., Petre, R., Soong, Y., Chan, K.-W., Lodha, G. S., Namba, Y., and Yu, J. (1998). Development of a multilayer supermirror for hard x-ray telescopes. In Hoover, R. B. and Walker, A. B., editors, *X-Ray Optics, Instruments, and Missions*, volume 3444 of *Society of Photo-Optical Instrumentation Engineers (SPIE) Conference Series*, pages 569–575.

[Telleschi et al., 2005] Telleschi, A., Güdel, M., Briggs, K., Audard, M., Ness, J.-U., and Skinner, S. L. (2005). Coronal Evolution of the Sun in Time: High-Resolution X-Ray Spectroscopy of Solar Analogs with Different Ages. *Astrophys. J.*, 622:653–679.

[The Lynx Team, 2018] The Lynx Team (2018). The Lynx Mission Concept Study Interim Report. *arXiv e-prints*, page arXiv:1809.09642.

[Thole, 1973] Thole, J. M. (1973). *The OSO-7 Mission*, page 7.

[Thornton and Hoffman, 1989] Thornton, J. A. and Hoffman, D. (1989). Stress-related effects in thin films. *Thin Solid Films*, 171(1):5 – 31.

[Tiwari et al., 2012] Tiwari, M. . K., Gupta, P., Sinha, A. K., Garg, C. K., Singh, A. K., Kane, S. R., Garg, S. R., and Lodha, G. S. (2012). Commissioning of a microprobe-xrf beamline (bl-16) on indus-2 synchrotron source. *AIP Conference Proceedings*, 1447(1):499–500.

[Truemper, 1982] Truemper, J. (1982). The ROSAT mission. *Advances in Space Research*, 2:241–249.

[Tsunemi et al., 1986] Tsunemi, H., Yamashita, K., Masai, K., Hayakawa, S., and Koyama, K. (1986). X-ray spectra of the Cassiopeia A and TYCHO supernova remnants and their element abundances. *Astrophys. J.*, 306:248–254.

[Tucker et al., 1998] Tucker, W. H., David, L. P., and Pen, U. (1998). In Search of Killer Clusters: Cosmological Implications of the 1E0657-56, the Hottest Known Galaxy Cluster. In *American Astronomical Society Meeting Abstracts #192*, volume 192 of *American Astronomical Society Meeting Abstracts*, page 37.01.

[Turner et al., 1981] Turner, M. J. L., Smith, A., and Zimmermann, H. U. (1981). The medium energy instrument on EXOSAT. *Space Sci. Rev.*, 30:513–524.

[Turner et al., 1989] Turner, M. J. L., Thomas, H. D., Patchett, B. E., Reading, D. H., Makishima, K., Ohashi, T., Dotani, T., Hayashida, K., Inoue, H., Kondo, H., Koyama, K., Mitsusa, K., Ogawara, Y., Takano, S., Awaki, H., Tawara, Y., and Nakamura, N. (1989). The large area counter on Ginga. *Publications of the Astronomical Society of Japan*, 41:345–372.

[Vadawale et al., 2018] Vadawale, S. V., Chattopadhyay, T., Mithun, N. P. S., Rao, A. R., Bhattacharya, D., Vibhute, A., Bhalerao, V. B., Dewangan, G. C., Misra, R., Paul, B., Basu, A., Joshi, B. C., Sreekumar, S., Samuel, E., Priya, P., Vinod, P., and Seetha, S. (2018). Phase-resolved X-ray polarimetry of the Crab pulsar with the AstroSat CZT Imager. *Nature Astronomy*, 2:50–55.

[Vinogradov and Zeldovich, 1977] Vinogradov, A. V. and Zeldovich, B. Y. (1977). X-ray and far uv multilayer mirrors: Principles and possibilities. *Applied Optics*, 16:89–93.

[Weisskopf et al., 2010] Weisskopf, M. C., Elsner, R. F., and O'Dell, S. L. (2010). On understanding the figures of merit for detection and measurement of x-ray polarization. In *Space Telescopes and Instrumentation 2010: Ultraviolet to Gamma Ray*, volume 7732 of *Society of Photo-Optical Instrumentation Engineers (SPIE) Conference Series*, page 77320E.

[Weisskopf et al., 2016] Weisskopf, M. C., Ramsey, B., O'Dell, S. L., Tennant, A., Elsner, R., Soffita, P., Bellazzini, R., Costa, E., Kolodziejczak, J., Kaspi, V., Mulieri, F., Marshall, H., Matt, G., and Romani, R. (2016). The Imaging X-ray Polarimetry Explorer (IXPE). *Results in Physics*, 6:1179–1180.

[Weisskopf et al., 1978] Weisskopf, M. C., Silver, E. H., Kestenbaum, H. L., Long, K. S., and Novick, R. (1978). A precision measurement of the X-ray polarization of the Crab Nebula without pulsar contamination. *Astrophys. J.*, 220:L117–L121.

[Weisskopf et al., 2000] Weisskopf, M. C., Tananbaum, H. D., Van Speybroeck, L. P., and O'Dell, S. L. (2000). Chandra X-ray Observatory (CXO): overview. In Truemper, J. E. and Aschenbach, B., editors, *X-Ray Optics, Instruments, and Missions III*, volume 4012 of *Society of Photo-Optical Instrumentation Engineers (SPIE) Conference Series*, pages 2–16.

[Wells et al., 2004] Wells, A. A., Gehrels, N. A., White, N. E., Barthelmy, S. D., Nousek, J. A., Burrows, D. N., Roming, P. W. A., Mason, K. O., Chincarini, G., and Giommi, P. (2004). The SWIFT Gamma-Ray Burst Observatory. In Hasinger, G. and Turner, M. J. L., editors, *UV and Gamma-Ray Space Telescope Systems*, volume 5488 of *Society of Photo-Optical Instrumentation Engineers (SPIE) Conference Series*, pages 403–414.

[Windt, 1998] Windt, D. L. (1998). IMD–Software for modeling the optical properties of multilayer films. *Computers in Physics*, 12:360–370.

[Windt et al., 2004] Windt, D. L., Donguy, S., Seely, J. F., Kjornrattanawanich, B., Gullikson, E. M., Walton, C. C., Golub, L., and DeLuca, E. (2004). EUV multilayers for solar physics. In Citterio, O. and O'Dell, S. L., editors, *Optics for EUV, X-Ray, and Gamma-Ray Astronomy*, volume 5168 of *Society of Photo-Optical Instrumentation Engineers (SPIE) Conference Series*, pages 1–11.

[Wolter, 1952] Wolter, H. (1952). Spiegelsysteme streifenden Einfalls als abbildende Optiken fontgenstrahlen. *Annalen der Physik*, 445:94–114.

[Woltjer, 1964] Woltjer, L. (1964). X-Rays and Type I Supernova Remnants. *Astrophys. J.*, 140:1309–1313.

[Yadav et al., 2016] Yadav, J. S., Agrawal, P. C., Antia, H. M., Chauhan, J. V., Dedhia, D., Katoch, T., Madhwani, P., Manchanda, R. K., Misra, R., Pahari, M., Paul, B., and Shah, P. (2016). Large Area X-ray Proportional Counter (LAXPC) instrument onboard ASTROSAT. In *Space Telescopes and Instrumentation 2016: Ultraviolet to Gamma Ray*, volume 9905 of *Society of Photo-Optical Instrumentation Engineers (SPIE) Conference Series*, page 99051D.

[Yonetoku et al., 2011] Yonetoku, D., Murakami, T., Gunji, S., Mihara, T., Sakashita, T., Morihara, Y., Kikuchi, Y., Takahashi, T., Fujimoto, H., Toukairin, N., Kodama, Y., Kubo, S., and Ikaros Demonstration Team (2011). Gamma-Ray Burst Polarimeter (GAP) aboard the Small Solar Power Sail Demonstrator IKAROS. *Publications of the Astronomical Society of Japan*, 63:625.

[Zombeck et al., 1981] Zombeck, M. V., Wyman, C. C., and Weisskopf, M. C. (1981). High resolution X-ray scattering measurements for Advanced X-ray Astrophysics Facility /AXAF/. In Hunt, G. H., editor, *Radiation scattering in optical systems*, volume 257 of *Society of Photo-Optical Instrumentation Engineers (SPIE) Conference Series*, pages 230–247.

List of corrections

I have made the following corrections in the corrected copy of the thesis as per suggestions of the second examiner. List of all corrections incorporated in the thesis are detailed below.

1. **Comment**: Chapter-2 pg. 23, Eqn. No. 2.13, it is not clear whether constant number 69 is written in minute unit? Please also mention it in a correct manner along with proper reference.

   Response: The constant number 69 is in the units of minute. I have modified the equation to increase the clarity of the units. I have also provided a reference for that equation, Bass et al.2010.

2. **Comment**: In figure 2.5, please also mention text that represents the transmitted X-rat beam.

   Response: I have modified figure 2.5 mentioning the transmitted X-ray beam.

3. **Comment**: Chapter-2 pg. 28, mentioned density values make confusion in readability. Give a separation between numerical value and its unit. For example, it should be written as Nickel (Ni) (8.9 g/cc) rather than (8.9g/cc). Please make corrections at the other places as well.

   Response: I have changed the suggested correction in throughout the thesis. I have given a space gap between the number and the unit where ever needed.

4. **Comment**: Chapter-2 pg. 30, figure caption 2.8: 'nano-meter (nm)' should be written as 'nanometers (nm)'

   Response: I have changed 'nano-meters (nm)' as 'nanometers (nm)' in the figure caption 2.8.

5. **Comment**: Chapter-3 pg. 73, 'beam line 16' should be written at beamline (BL-16).

   Response: I have changed beam line 16 to eamline (BL-16)

6. **Comment**: At several places multilaye sample named W-B$_4$C on the other it is also mentioned in the form W/B$_4$C. Kindly ensure uniformity in the representation.

   Response: I have incorporated these modifications by keeping all the sample names in W/B$_4$C configuration.

7. **Comment**: Chapter-4 pg. 79, 'For e.g., by changing...' should be replaced with 'for example, by changing'.
   Response: I have changed the statement as per suggestion in page number 79.

8. **Comment**: On the same page, the sentence is not clear, 'So, the drop in reflectivity for the sample during the first 11 months is mainly due to the under sampling of the measurement data.' The corrections mark in the red color may improve the readability. Please make it as appropriate.

   Response: I have mention the above referred statement in the italic form to emphasize the the importance of the statement for better readability.

9. **Comment**: On the same page, 'the density of B$_4$C is 4.1 g/cc (bulk density is 2.52)'. Kindly ensure that the density value mentioned for the B$_4$C thin film medium is correct. It looks bit strange to me.

   Response: The density of B$_4$C has increased in the sample due to the interlayer diffusion with the W layer which is adjacent to it. Since the W density is very large compared to that B$_4$C, the overall density of B$_4$C layer has increased in the sample. We have obtained the density values by fitting the X-ray reflectivity data.

10. **Comment**: Chapter-5 pg. 141, Figure 5.19 is not properly visible.

    Response: I have replaced the figure with the higher resolution picture for better visibility.